Precepting Medical Residents in the Office

Edited by

Paul M Paulman, MD
Professor and Predoctoral Director
Department of Family Medicine
University of Nebraska College of Medicine

Audrey A Paulman, MD, MMM
Clinical Assistant Professor
Department of Family Medicine
University of Nebraska College of Medicine

Jeffrey D Harrison, MD
Associate Professor and Residency Director
Department of Family Medicine
University of Nebraska College of Medicine

Jeffrey L Susman, MD
Professor and Chair
Department of Family Medicine
University of Cincinnati

and

Kate Finkelstein, MLIS
Government Relations Senior Associate
DeBrunner & Associates

Radcliffe Publishing
Oxford • Seattle

Radcliffe Publishing Ltd
18 Marcham Road
Abingdon
Oxon OX14 1AA
United Kingdom

www.radcliffe-oxford.com
Electronic catalogue and worldwide online ordering facility.

British Library Cataloguing in Publication Data

A catalogue record for this book is available from the British Library.

ISBN-10: 1 84619 102 5
ISBN-13: 978 184619 102 2

Typeset by Aarontype Ltd, Easton, Bristol, UK
Printed and bound by TJ International Ltd, Padstow, Cornwall, UK

Contents

Foreword

Most readers are familiar with the phrase 'the secret of the care of the patient is in caring for the patient', the final line of Peabody's seminal article on patient care published in the *Journal of the American Medical Association* (19 March 1927).

However, some of his other observations, on medical trainees, earlier in the same article have been mostly forgotten.

The most common criticism made at present by older practitioners is that young graduates have been taught a great deal about the mechanism of disease, but very little about the practice of medicine – or, to put it more bluntly, they are too 'scientific' and do not know how to take care of patients.

recent graduates, who find that in the actual practice of medicine they encounter many situations which they had not been led to anticipate and which they are not prepared to meet effectively.

And while they have been absorbed in the difficult task of digesting and correlating new knowledge, it has been easy to overlook the fact that the application of the principles of science to the diagnosis and treatment of disease is only one limited aspect of medical practice. The practice of medicine in its broadest sense includes the whole relationship of the physician with his patient. It is an art, based to an increasing extent on the medical sciences, but comprising much that still remains outside the realm of any science ...

Interesting, isn't it? Another example of the more things change, the more they stay the same.

Today we talk about imparting knowledge, skills and attitude and, for most people, this represents a continual learning process for both trainer and trainee. In his first book, *Precepting Medical Students in the Office*, Dr Paulman and his fellow authors did a commendable job in producing a comprehensive handbook for community preceptors with medical students in the office-based setting. In this, the second book, he lends his knowledge and skills to the issues of precepting medical residents in the ambulatory setting, again producing a comprehensive handbook for precepting residents.

Although modern technology can change the way in which students acquire knowledge and, in some cases, skills, there is no substitute for a true mentor. In Greek mythology, Mentor was the friend of Odysseus who was entrusted with the education of Odysseus' son, Telemachus. Webster's dictionary defines a mentor as 'a trusted counselor or guide.' In medicine, perhaps more than in any other profession, our mentors have always enjoyed a special place in our hearts and minds. In reciting the Hippocratic oath, new physicians pledge to 'keep this, my oath and covenant, to regard him who teaches this art equally with my parents.' Although some professional athletes may contend that 'I am not a role model', there is no doubt where you and I, as preceptors, stand on this issue. We *are* role models. We *are* mentors and upon us falls the responsibility to prepare tomorrow's physicians for careers in public service that we can only begin to comprehend.

James Stageman, MD
Associate Professor, Department of Family Medicine
University of Nebraska College of Medicine
Assistant Dean, University of Nebraska College of Medicine
May 2006

Preface

This book has been produced to serve as a resource for community physicians who bring medical residents into their practices and train them in their offices. As hospital stays decrease in length and as more patient care is moved to the ambulatory setting, there is an increasing need for community-based training for medical residents in a variety of specialties.

The contributors have been recruited from the ranks of community teaching physicians and community- and university-based residency educators in family medicine, internal medicine and pediatrics. This book has been designed with the busy community physician in mind, and each chapter is intended to serve as a practical, concise, easily read, stand-alone resource on the topic covered. Those who read the entire volume will note differences in the writing styles in the various chapters and a certain redundancy with regard to key topics and issues. These are both inevitable in this type of educational manual.

The editors would like to dedicate this book to all of the community physicians who give of their time, talents and resources to train medical residents in their offices.

Paul M Paulman
Audrey A Paulman
Jeffrey D Harrison
Jeffrey L Susman
Kate Finkelstein
May 2006

About the Editors

Paul M Paulman, MD
Professor and Predoctoral Director
Department of Family Medicine
University of Nebraska College of Medicine, Omaha, NE

Audrey A Paulman, MD, MMM
Clinical Assistant Professor
Department of Family Medicine
University of Nebraska College of Medicine, Omaha, NE

Jeffrey D Harrison, MD
Associate Professor and Residency Director
Department of Family Medicine
University of Nebraska College of Medicine, Omaha, NE

Jeffrey L Susman, MD
Professor and Chair
Department of Family Medicine
University of Cincinnati, Cincinnati, OH

Kate Finkelstein, MLIS
Government Relations Senior Associate
DeBrunner & Associates, Sterling, VA

List of Contributors

Dale R Agner, MD
Commander 42nd Medical Operations Squadron
US Air Force – Maxwell Air Force Base

Dennis Baker, PhD
Assistant Dean for Faculty Development
Florida State University College of Medicine, Tallahassee, FL

Dan Benzie, MD
President
Gateway Family Health Clinic, Moose Lake, MN

Kaye Carstens, MD
Associate Professor
Nebraska Medical Center, Omaha, NE

Alexander W Chessman, MD
Professor
Department of Family Medicine, University of South Carolina, Charleston, SC

Deborah S Clements, MD, FAAFP
Associate Program Director
University of Kansas Medical Center, Kansas City, KS

Brian Finley, MD
Associate Professor
Nebraska Medical Center, Omaha, NE

Richard Fruehling, MD
Assistant Professor
Nebraska Medical Center, Grand Island, NE

Michael R Gloor, FACHE
President and CEO
Saint Francis Medical Center, Grand Island, NE

Karla Hemesath, PhD
Director of Curriculum and Evaluation
Aurora Health Care, Madison Fam Prac Res, Milwaukee, WI

Jeffrey W Hill, MD
Associate Professor
Nebraska Medical Center, Omaha, NE

Michael Horn, MD
Vice President for Medical Affairs
Saint Francis Medical Center, Grand Island, NE

Stanley M Kozakowski, MD
Director
Family Medicine Residency Program, Hunterdon Medical Center, Flemington, NJ

Alan Lembitz, MD
Vice President
COPIC Companies, Denver, CO

Amy L Longo, JD
Adjunct Asst Professor, Preventive and Societal Medicine
University of Nebraska College of Medicine, Omaha, NE

Mary Ann Manners, MSPH
Instructor
Nebraska Medical Center, Omaha, NE

Fred McCurdy, MD
Professor and Regional Chairman
Department of Pediatrics, Texas Tech Medical Center, Amarillo, TX

David V O'Dell, MD
Associate Professor and Director of Primary Care
Nebraska Medical Center, Omaha, NE

Kenneth G Reinert, MD
US Air Force – Scott Air Force Base

Edward Shahady, MD
Director, Diabetes Master Clinician Program
Florida Academy of Family Physicians Foundation, Jacksonville, FL

Kent Sheets, PhD
Associate Professor and Director of Educational Development
Department of Family Medicine, University of Michigan, Ann Arbor, MI

Eric Skye, MD
Assistant Professor
Department of Family Medicine, University of Michigan, Ann Arbor, MI

Jeffrey A Stearns, MD
Associate Dean
University of Wisconsin Medical School, Milwaukee, WI

David Steele, PhD
Professor of Family Medicine and Rural Health
Florida State University College of Medicine, Tallahassee, FL

Marian R Stuart, PhD
Clinical Professor of Family Medicine and Director of Behavioral Science
Department of Family Medicine, Robert Wood Johnson Medical School,
New Brunswick, NJ

Section I

The Resident and Teaching Techniques

Chapter 1

Value of Office-Based Teaching

Deborah S Clements, MD, FAAFP

Key Points

- Office-based teaching of medical residents offers residents invaluable learning experiences.
- The knowledge and skills acquired by medical residents in the community preceptor's office cannot be acquired in other venues.

The importance of community training of medical residents cannot be over-emphasized. During the late 1890s, Osler anticipated the eventual separation of traditional hospital-based teaching and the realities of community-based practice and ambulatory models of care.

In his book, *Time to Heal*, Kenneth Ludmerer states, 'Community-based teaching of medicine provides every student with an opportunity to learn and know clinical medicine as it is practiced today and to meet and learn about patients, their lives, their communities and their doctors.' Nowhere is this more evident than in community-based residency training of physicians. The contributions of thousands of community physicians to the education of medical residents are critical in introducing useful practice models in an environment that closely approximates the typical practice of medicine, and in encouraging residents to develop their own practice style, to seek the setting most appropriate for their personal and professional fulfillment, and to provide role models and mentors for young physicians. Through sustained interactions with community faculty, residents gain an appreciation of the vital relationships among physicians across specialties, patients and their communities.

Academic health centers affiliated with community faculty realize many benefits as a direct result of their combined efforts, including closer ties with physicians in the community, increased opportunities to collaborate in practice-based research, more comprehensive faculty development, and revenue generated from patient referrals.

Undeniably, changes in the provision of medical care in the US over the past decade have presented some challenges to all medical educators. Scientific knowledge, diagnostic tools and treatment modalities have expanded dramatically, resulting in a far more extensive curriculum for residency training. As payment systems moved from fee-for-service to third-party administration models, the measurement of successful clinical education began to focus increasingly on profitability and penetration of the market. Improvements in treatment combined with economic pressures resulted in shorter inpatient stays, and a shift of patient care to the ambulatory clinic. Increased regulatory pressures have shifted attention to the business of medicine, sometimes at the expense of the art and science of medicine. Finally, electronic access to information has changed the landscape of the patient–physician interaction, placing a renewed emphasis on the need for community physicians to manage relationships and knowledge in addition to providing medical skills.

Despite these challenges, community physicians remain satisfied with their career choice and continue their commitment to their patients and communities. Physician preceptors appreciate the adage that teaching is learning twice, using their interactions with residents both to improve their own understanding and to impart to their learners a full appreciation of longitudinal care, exacerbation of chronic conditions, the importance of a therapeutic alliance and the impact of the patient's family, work and community on the patient's health.

Through their work with community physicians, residents also develop the ability to effectively and safely manage uncertainty, to function as a member of a healthcare team and to integrate community resources into the optimal care of their patients.

According to Ludmerer, the power of medical education in the academic health center is limited, particularly with regard to its ability to produce doctors who are caring, socially responsible, and capable of behaving as patient advocates in all practice environments. It is important to recognize that the caliber of doctors we have represents a negotiation between medical education and society. That negotiation is successful in large part because of the efforts of community physician educators.

Chapter 2

Identifying Learning Needs of Residents

Mary Ann Manners, MSPH

Key Points

- Residency is the *application* and, most importantly, *problem-solving* part of previous undergraduate medical learning.
- Adjusting your teaching to the resident's learning needs can enhance the educational experience for the resident and preceptor.
- The preceptor's office offers unique learning opportunities for residents at all stages of training and from all backgrounds.

Introduction

Each medical graduate comes into residency with different knowledge bases, clinical experiences, fears, attitudes and, most obviously, strengths and weaknesses. A primary emphasis of undergraduate medical education is on mountains of memorization: anatomy and physiology, pharmacology, signs, symptoms and diagnoses, along with manual techniques of physical and laboratory examinations. Although problem-based learning (PBL) and clinical rotations offer some hands-on application, students have little primary responsibility. Residency provides the opportunity to fine-tune the graduate's knowledge and techniques within the context of a variety of patient care possibilities. Thus, in educational terms, residency is the *application*, and most importantly, the *problem-solving* part of previous undergraduate medical learning. Perhaps the prime benefit of residency is the guided tour that experienced physicians provide in the application of medical knowledge during the numerous rotations – when, where, why and how with the young and old, male and female, a variety of presentations, differing circumstances and concurrent diseases. Specifically, learning the 'in-the-trenches' techniques that experienced physicians offer of the knowledge, application and problem solving in your specialty is the goal for residents rotating through your office.

Keeping this cumulative progression of medical education in mind, the experiences and needs of residents rotating to your office will be more apparent. Even with advances in technology, physicians are more than technicians. More than the textbook descriptions, residents need to learn how to apply the vast amounts of knowledge that they possess – which symptom or test is more valuable in certain circumstances, how to prioritize problems, the 'red flags' of the rare versus the common, and what laboratory tests provide the most fruitful results. In addition, they face the huge area of patient interactions, continuity, interview skills, prevention and patient education, along with behavior changes. Moreover, each specialty has manual techniques and procedures that can be honed beyond what is learned in undergraduate training. You are uniquely able to provide the application and problem-solving parts of medicine. Since residents are not usually competing with another student or resident for patients, the one-to-one time is maximized.

This chapter cannot address all the various content areas of each specialty. It will specifically address the types of exposures and processes needed by residents in the private office settings, by the year of residency. Although there is overlap from year to year, and specific residents may be ahead or behind in their personal level of education, the benefit *and* the challenge of individualizing your educational efforts are limitless in a private practice setting.

A Word About Non-Traditional Residents

Each year there are a few more non-traditional medical students, who then advance to residency. The non-traditional residents are older, have changed careers, or may have military experience. These residents bring a lot to the table, and are generally a wonderful influence on cohorts. They are commonly grounded in real-world experiences, more mature, more confident, and can see the big picture. They have positive attitudes, are able to put things in perspective, are serious about responsibilities, and 'look the part' of a physician, so are easily accepted by patients. Often they have had some experience of the healthcare system, either personally or through their family, which is a reference point for what kind of physician they want to become, and they are willing to work hard to get there. Educationally, they are self-motivated and eager to learn as much as they can. Frequently they are more comfortable in their own skin, and find it easier to admit what they don't know, to ask for help, or even to request additional resources, and extra clinical learning opportunities.

However, *some* of these non-traditional residents have difficulty in other areas, which aren't quite as apparent in the traditional residents. They may have experienced a drastic change and sacrifice in their lifestyle in order to enter medical school. Balancing the time demands of a spouse and children with hours on call, weekend duties, etc., may be more difficult. Worries about decreased income and mounting debt may increase excess moonlighting. They may struggle with the extended lack of autonomy and independence. Some don't like activities that they perceive as 'a waste of time' – they want to be finished and get their ticket stamped. In a few instances, these residents may appear rigid, try to cover up deficiencies, convey an attitude of already knowing everything, and thus are not very 'teachable.' As attendings and faculty, it is also easy to accept non-traditional residents who appear and act in a more mature manner as a colleague, to assume that they know more than they have proven, and to ignore behavior that would not be accepted in a younger resident.

The majority of the time, non-traditional residents are eager learners, a delight to have in a practice, and contribute much. However, educators need to keep alert for any problematic situations. Medical education in a private office has a great ability to individualize the one-on-one time spent with resident physicians, and to take all of these factors into consideration, if watched carefully. Subtle changes in teaching approaches can usually address these differences.

First-Year Residents/Interns

The internship year is primarily the *application* phase of their undergraduate education – learning what to do with all that memorized information. Since each medical school curriculum is slightly different, each graduate has a unique foundation of strengths, skills, attitudes and weaknesses or gaps in education and experience. One's natural inclination is to assume a certain breadth of knowledge based on personal experiences, or on preceding residents who have been on a rotation. Although tempting, this sets up a first-year resident for expectations that may or may not be realistic, often through no fault of the resident.

First-year residents are in a unique situation. They are excited about jumping in and learning, but their anxiety is high because of the increased responsibility for patient care. They are working with other residents who have come from various different medical schools, and they worry about how they will measure up. Like medical school, each month brings a different rotation – just when they feel comfortable with one team, the whole process starts again. And they are well aware that each attending physician has his or her own style, office procedures, staff preference and attitudes, etc.

You may not see first-year residents in your private offices, as most of the internship year is spent in hospital-based rotations. This formative year is important for laying the groundwork for the following years.

Questions and Needs

Orientation to Your Practice (see Chapter 6)

Relieving some anxiety early on can set the stage for residents to maximize learning. This includes introductions to personnel, administrative practices, community, special opportunities, expectations, call schedule, and internal and outside resources. Questions may include the following. Are there any patients they may not see? Are they expected to cover for emergencies? For nursing homes? For school sports physicals or classroom or presentations? For phone triage?

Resident Supervision in Your Practice (see Chapter 7)

Will they observe? Will they interview and present? Will they see as a team? Will they interview and examine? Will you see all patients with residents? If so, for how long? Or do you have residents present cases only for approval before the patient leaves the office? Do you supervise prescriptions? Laboratory orders? Billing?

Baseline Assessment

Each resident's knowledge base, psychomotor skills and techniques, communication skills, attitude, confidence, responsibility and work ethic are determined by the preceptor at baseline. This can be done through a series of interviews and/ or observations over the first week, as the resident relaxes. Helpful points include what experience this resident has had with different age groups, genders, specific procedures and specialties. Each resident has specific wants or needs of the learning expectations on this rotation.

Setting a Positive Attitude and Atmosphere for Learning

It is of utmost importance that you let residents know you expect them to have a variety of experiences, with some strengths, gaps and/or weaknesses. However, in order to fill in the gaps you first need to know what they are. It is helpful to normalize the process of recognizing strengths and weaknesses, the process of filling in gaps and aiding each other, as colleagues. It can actually be dangerous to 'cover' areas of weakness. Questioning or asking for help is a sign of responsibility and maturity. In a world of lifelong learning, this will be essential not just for residency, but for all their practicing years, for patient interactions, and future practice partners. The format is set to review errors and learn from them (e.g. activities such as morbidity and mortality conferences).

Medical Foundation of Your Practice

Initial cases usually cover the basics of your specialty, the 10 to 15 most common things you see in your office, including:

- a demonstration of the specific exam techniques, skills and acceptable variations, patient presentations and symptoms
- a variety of ages, genders, socio-economic groups and personalities
- common treatments, dosages, laboratory tests, etc.
- a discussion of your particular style of practice – how to handle interactions with you, nurses and other allied professionals, patient education, behavior change, discussion of side-effects, dangers of a specific procedure, informed consent, etc.

You (a Role Model)

A 'particular strength of the (private practice) experience may be the frequent and effective resident–preceptor interactions'.[1] The preceptor needs to be physically present, approachable, and have time for consulting when asked. Unless there are several residents in a practice at one time, interns will not have a senior resident to consult, which is a model they have learned in hospital rotations. The attending is the final source of information for the intern. Their knowledge is expanded with gentle probing. For example, what would you change if this patient was 65? Or if they were 25? Or if they were a child? Or if they had high blood pressure? Or if they had no insurance? In addition, attitude and approach to patients will be observed and learned as much as or more than anything that comes from the preceptor's mouth.

Time

The first-year resident needs time – time to manage all the details, time to interact with numerous office personnel and community agencies, to make referrals, to look up problems or treatments in reference books, to reflect, consult, and research areas of weakness. In addition, the intern will review charts and patients at the end of the day, including what was done, what still needs to be done, plans for follow-up, any questions after the fact, etc. *The first year of residency is not the time to push time efficiency.* Thoroughness comes first.

Feedback

Interns will be lacking confidence in their ability to handle cases well, make the right assessments, interact smoothly, chart correctly, etc. For all these things and more they will need recognition of their successes in order to boost their self-confidence and address their fear of doing something wrong. In order to grow, they need constructive suggestions on ways to improve (*see* Chapter 1).

Second-Year Residents

Second-year residents have usually worked through many of the differences arising from their various backgrounds, are increasing in self-confidence, and are ready to be more independent. However, most of their experience up to this time has been of inpatient medicine. The private practice setting will provide the opportunity 'to put the tertiary care experience of internship in the broader perspective . . .'.[2] While continuing to learn applications, this is the opportunity to seriously begin the more difficult *problem-solving* aspect of education. Hopefully, the second-year resident will be more comfortable discussing their personal strengths and weaknesses and their goals for the rotation. A mutual agreement is developed to address their needs and wants along with the preceptors' objectives. The R2 year also introduces the possibility of residents teaching other students or even first-year residents if there are both in the practice at the same time. Teaching others becomes a responsibility in the second year of residency.

Needs of R2 Residents

Orientation and Baseline Assessments

See above for first-year residents.

Increased Responsibility and Independence

Second-year residents were closely supervised during the intern year. More responsibility will now be taken, with the R2 making more of their own decisions, at least initially. Once assessment has demonstrated the knowledge, skills and attitudes of the R2, preferences for supervision may allow more or less direct supervision by the preceptor. Mentoring is helpful, when possible, allowing the resident the responsibility of discussing difficult situations, diagnoses, unsuccessful outcomes, etc. with patients and their families.

Opportunity to Teach Others

If there are students, interns or even other professionals in the office, you could allow the second-year resident to take someone 'under their wing' and assist in teaching.

Exposure to a Balance of Personal and Professional Activities

Effective precepting involves showing that practice involves more than just clinical and inpatient time, and demonstrating how to prioritize other activities, scheduling personal and family time, time for continuing education, etc. Including the resident in these activities can be an eye-opener to him or her.

Informal Discussions

Current 'hot topics', medical ethics, 'war stories' and words of wisdom related to cases of the day, as well as unofficial 'morbidity and mortality' discussions, are helpful.

Beginning to Focus on Time Efficiency

The schedule can begin to allow more patients, with continuity when possible, with a variety of problems.

Role Models

Telling someone how to act, what to think, and the necessary values or attitudes rarely works as effectively as seeing these in action. Attitudes, style, approach, techniques, patient education, suggestions for behavior change, listening and personal experience speak volumes to the R2.

Feedback

This involves positive and constructive suggestions specific to their level of education and work (*see* Chapter 6)

Upper-Level Residents

Upper-level residents past their second year of training need to expand their learning in all directions, with the anticipation of a private practice. On the brink of becoming completely autonomous, upper-level residents need to feel that they possess the skills necessary to take this leap, including thorough and extensive medical skills in the office and hospital, and in business aspects of practice, as well as professional and personal balance. Many third- and fourth-year rotations are electives, indicating that the residents have specific educational areas which they want or need to expand. At this stage, educational efforts need to focus on the residents' perceived needs, together with the highest level of *problem solving* for your specialty, along with the nuts and bolts of private practice, and being a physician in a community.

Residents during these years actually start to collect items that they wish to use in practice, and may have taken for granted through the years. Items such as new patient questionnaires, sample chart forms, educational models, billing forms, patient education brochures and even specific reference books seem more important. This is the very tangible facet of residency, because the end is in sight. Keeping education focused on their educational needs and wants, and very applicable, can reduce the 'senioritis' that may rear its head at this stage.

Upper-Level Residents' Needs

Orientation and Assessment

The focus is on the needs and wants of the resident, which may form a very specific list.

Junior Colleague Status

There is a need for increased autonomy, less supervision, more responsibility, larger patient load time and efficient patient care.

Challenging Patients

These residents need to see the entire breadth of practice – all the nitty-gritty, problematic patients – in order to address a high level of problem-solving situations, including:

- complex, multi-problem patients, unusual presentations, treatment failures
- difficult patients (e.g. angry, manipulative, ethnic-minority or non-English-speaking patients)
- reliable medical referral sources, community agencies and others
- occupational health, relative to your practice demographics and location
- dysfunctional families, and family conferences.

Teaching and Leadership Roles

- Medical students, R1 residents, other health profession students.
- Conflict resolution among team members and staff.

Business and Practical Aspects of Medical Practice (see *Chapter 12 for more details*)

These include:

- scheduling, phone triage, billing and collections
- personnel management, hiring, firing and vacations
- influence of insurance, Medicare, Medicaid and other programs on your practice
- record-keeping and charting systems, patient surveys, educational models and brochures.

Informal Personal Discussions

These include:

- practice site selection, selection process, advantages and disadvantages of multi-specialty groups, specialty-specific practices, what to avoid, signing bonuses, 'head hunters', etc.
- words of wisdom and/or tales of caution about contracts, partnerships and shared facilities
- finance – how to choose personal resources and experts (e.g. attorney, financial planner, banker, insurance agent)
- specialty board preparation – suggestions and recommendations, articles, areas of interest, unexpected or problematic topics, etc.

Role Modeling

In addition to areas previously covered, at least engaging residents in discussion of, but preferably involving them in the following activities:

- ethical dilemmas, medical mistakes (*see* Chapter 9)
- professional activities – continuing education, professional organizations, medical society/hospital meetings, boards, etc.
- community service – schools, under-served communities, sports, altruistic/charitable organizations.

Conclusion

The private office is a wonderful component of resident education, which allows the resident to view the perspective of complete practice possibilities, gaining insight from experienced professionals, and obtaining the skills to pass boards and become an independent physician in the community. It offers:

1 a better mix of patients with regard to social class and spectrum of medical problems
2 more continuity of care
3 a greater opportunity for resident–preceptor interactions
4 more responsibility for patients.[1]

Private practitioners can provide the best of 'apprentice'-style education, tailoring their one-to-one efforts to the educational needs of each resident. A preceptor provides the breadth of medical teaching along with significant personal role modeling that allows the resident to envision him- or herself in practice.

References

1 Napodano RJ, Schuster BL, Krackov SK *et al*. (1984) Use of private offices in education of residents in internal medicine. *Arch Intern Med.* **2:** 303–5.
2 Philbrick JT, Connelly JE, Corbett EC Jr *et al*. (1990) Restoring balance to internal medicine training: the case for the teaching office practice. *Am J Med Sci.* **1:** 43–9.

Further reading

Victor LD (1994) *The Residency Handbook.* Parthenon Publishing Group, New York.
Whitman N and Schwenk TL (1995) *Preceptors as Teachers: A Guide to Clinical Teaching.* University of Utah School of Medicine, Salt Lake City, UT.

Chapter 3

Creating the Learning Environment

Fred McCurdy, MD

Key Points

- A learning contract between the preceptor and the resident can contribute to an effective learning environment.
- A preceptor models lifelong learning habits.

Creating the Learning Environment

Basic objectives are organized in three general areas: patient-centered, office-centered, and physician-centered. A learning environment is created for all three areas. Students (this includes residents) must be motivated to learn, must be open-minded about the possibility that they can learn something new, and must possess some level of self-directed learning skill. By virtue of the fact that a preceptor is a self-directed, continuous learner, there is modeling of all of these behaviors for the resident. The learning process is facilitated by paying attention to the items discussed below.

- **Respect the learner**. Recognize the various stressors present (new experience, career decisions that the residents might be forced to make prematurely). Express belief that the resident is a valuable member of the team and is contributing to healthcare outcomes. Make a commitment to teaching visible by being positive about the resident being in the practice, acknowledging personal limits of knowledge, and setting realistic goals for the resident. A key point is that the preceptor can learn from the resident, and that a teacher is also a learner.
- **Value time.** Time is valuable, and effective time management is critical to professional and personal success for the preceptor and the resident.
- **Control the physical and social office environment.** The office is prepared to promote learning by briefing the office staff as well as the patients. In addition, the resident needs space to work and access to records, journals, books and computers.
- **Understand the impact of good teaching skills.** Relevant learning experiences are best (e.g. an emphasis on longitudinal care, dealing with people rather than cases or diseases, the impact of social and societal factors on patient health outcomes, emphasizing team-based care).

- **Negotiate a learning contract.** There is a need to establish some mutually agreed goals – a 'learning contract.' This contract of goals considers the resident's previous experiences and special skills, and assesses current knowledge so that it will tailor the residency to match these previous experiences. Direct observation of the resident working with patients may be needed to assess overall abilities to perform various tasks (e.g. taking a history, performing a physical examination, etc.). The learning contract must also support the resident by establishing a system to monitor for any situation that may cause harm to either the resident or your patient(s).
- **Promote professional behavior.** Model behaviors that illustrate the concepts of professionalism – caring, compassion, integrity and altruism – through coaching learners by rehearsing before, attending during the student–patient interaction and conversing with the student after the experience.
- **Continually assess learning.** Establish an appropriate level of responsibility using a graduated approach to give the resident more responsibility to demonstrate their capacity to take on additional responsibility. It is fine to trust gut feeling as you initially work with the resident. Feedback from patients, staff and others on how the resident is performing is helpful. Ask the resident to form an independent assessment and plan as part of the care of patients. Goal-related feedback is given at regular intervals, with written and oral summaries (summative evaluations) at specified points. This provides the resident with the opportunity to reflect on personal experience (self-assessment of the experience).

Creating a productive learning environment for a resident can require some work. The resident will be grateful for all of the efforts and they will learn a great deal about the actual practice of medicine. This can then be a tremendously powerful experience for the teacher and learner as both of them grow professionally.

Chapter 4

Matching Teaching and Learning Styles

Dan Benzie, MD

> **Key Points**
>
> - In order to enhance your residents' learning experience:
>   - determine your teaching style
>   - assess the residents' learning styles
>   - agree on the intended outcomes
>   - create a quality learning experience.

Teacher's Self-Assessment

Your preferred teaching styles may be based on past learning experiences, patient encounters, or teaching other students and residents. Each resident will have unique needs and backgrounds and the learning environment will vary significantly, so you will need to use a variety of teaching methods. There are a number of core attributes exhibited by community faculty. Excellent clinical teachers have been defined as those who are creative in their teaching styles and are:

- supportive and respectful of students and patients
- alert for opportunities to provide appropriate role modeling
- enthusiastic about their clinical practice and teaching.

As you prepare for a day of office teaching, consciously think of how you are going to interact with patients, what teaching techniques you intend to use, and what you hope to accomplish for yourself, the resident and your patients.

Review the Intended Outcomes

Keep good communication with your regional residency program so that you understand the goals and objectives for residents at different levels of training (these are listed in Chapter 2). Community teachers are encouraged to find out what knowledge, skills or attitudes should be focused on during the preceptorship, to take into account the resident's individual goals, and then to determine what outcomes can be expected from the preceptorship.

Help the resident to recognize the difference between a community practice and an academic training center. As well as the unusual and 'interesting' patients, the teaching should still focus on common clinical diagnoses and problems encountered in a community practice, including general principles of prevention, and the management of chronic health problems.

Attitudes that it is helpful to incorporate in your teaching efforts include professionalism, which is demonstrated through each physician's attitude toward patients, the healthcare team members and residents. The preceptorship also gives you an opportunity to incorporate teaching related to the ethical dilemmas that are part of daily practice.

Teaching Styles

Various styles of teaching should be used to meet the needs of different residents and in different situations. They include the following.

- **Assertive style.** The preceptor provides the information, such as providing a drug dosage or showing an appropriate method for holding the endoscope.
- **Suggestive style.** The alternatives are presented for the resident. This involves the sharing of your 'war stories', such as alternatives for hypertension management.
- **Collaborative style.** Residents are encouraged to do more problem solving. This style might include presenting the differential diagnosis for a patient with a headache or assessing the impact of the patient's lifestyle on the current health problem.
- **Facilitative style.** This is designed to promote more self-understanding by the resident. This is particularly helpful for teaching attitudes and emotions, such as delivering bad news to a patient or family.

A variety of different types of questions can be used to stimulate the resident's acquisition of knowledge. These include the following.

- **Factual questions** can be helpful for quickly assessing the resident's specific knowledge base. For example, 'What is the commonest cause of pancreatitis?'.
- **Broadening questions** attempt to enlarge the differential diagnosis for a current problem and may involve a review of the general management of an acute problem. For example, 'What else could cause this patient's pain?'.
- **Justifying questions** involve asking about specific treatment plans or medication side-effects, and will help you to determine the depth of the resident's understanding. For example, 'Why did you choose a diuretic to treat this patient?'.
- **Hypothetical questions** can help to utilize a single clinical encounter to assess other areas of the resident's knowledge. This technique can be applied by rephrasing questions so as to change the age or gender of the patient or the specifics of the complaint. For example, 'How would you treat bronchospasm if this patient were an infant?'.
- **Alternative questions** can be useful for helping residents to recognize that there are many correct ways of treating patients, and these questions are also helpful when reviewing the natural history of the disease process. For example, 'What else could you use to treat this patient's headache?'.

By using the various types of questions and teaching styles noted above, you can adapt the way you teach so that it is most appropriate to your resident's needs as well as to the intended teaching goal.

Residents' Learning Styles

Learning styles can range from dependent to independent, from avoidant to participant, and from competitive to collaborative. As medical students, residents have been motivated to outperform others by utilizing tests and grades. They should now begin the transition towards a more collaborative style where they can share ideas with patients, other residents and teachers. This collaboration will help them to develop group skills and improve teamwork. While some residents will have used avoidant styles to prevent them from becoming overwhelmed and anxious, others will demonstrate a more participative style as they contribute both to their own learning process and to that of others.

Resident physicians need to continue to enhance their clinical skills through-out their training. The community practice is the ideal location for the transition from preceptorship or dependent-style training to an apprenticeship or independent model.

Incorporated in the teaching are patient–physician communication skills (refined history taking), physical examination skills, problem solving (utilizing resources unique to your particular community) and principles of performing procedures. As many others have observed, this is an opportunity to assist the progression of the learner from the state of unconsciously incompetent to the

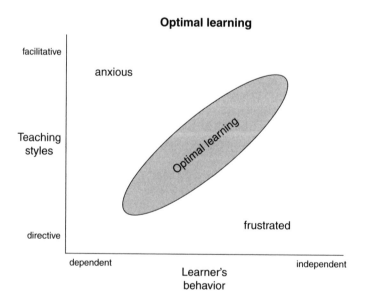

Figure 4.1 Matching teaching strategies and resident abilities to create an optimal learning climate. A first-year resident will benefit from dependent strategies in order to avoid anxiety, while a senior resident would benefit from more independent strategies to avoid frustration.

Table 4.1 Matching Learner Types and Teaching Strategies

Type of learner	Characteristics of learner	Teaching strategies
Independent	Seeks own goals and objectives; limited advice seeking; can be overly confident	Allow learner to set appropriate goals and objectives. Negotiate boundaries ahead of time (e.g. 'I want to be called with every admission to the inpatient service'). Foster insight when assistance or collaboration are needed
Visual	Learns best by seeing; may need mental picture in order to successfully complete task	Liberally use demonstrations, models and figures. Do not just discuss, but also demonstrate (e.g. 'Now, let me demonstrate how I do a mattress suture on this pig's foot')
Competitive	Every encounter is a chance to impress or obtain advantage; in extreme cases may foster conflict; often highly motivated	Channel motivation and activity appropriately. Reinforce positive behaviors and set clear expectations (e.g. 'My expectation is that the success of this rotation will be based on the success of all the residents here with us – being able to work effectively as a team member is part of this responsibility'). Encourage group and collaborative activities
Dependent or passive	May be unwilling to take the lead or go beyond clear boundaries; may appear to be less prepared or motivated	Work from areas of interest and strength. Foster greater self-reliance and determination. Set up non-threatening challenges (e.g. 'Why don't you go over to the hospital and do the history and physical examination on the patient with asthma and write initial orders?')
Auditory	Attuned to auditory learning; often will need to process information by reading or hearing it	Supplement office experience with readings, audiotapes and impromptu lectures (e.g. 'Let's now discuss the three important goals for diabetes care in this patient')
Collaborative	Enjoys working in collegial relationships; may be very relationship oriented; works well in teams	Encourage sharing of ideas and personal philosophy. Involve other members of the team. Solicit learner's input (e.g. 'So let's talk about the options for therapy of Ms Jones' hypertension')

state of consciously incompetent through consciously competent and finally to the performance of procedures while unconsciously competent.

Although residents' individual learning styles will vary significantly, you may use the learning opportunity to introduce new methods that are unique to the community practice or to your own experience. Different residents or circumstances will require that you modify these methods. Potential teaching/learning methods that the teacher should include are as follows:

- Socratic case presentations that may be incorporated into a morning report, hospital rounds, or observed patient–resident interactions in the office
- independent study, including textbooks, CD-ROM or the Internet
- experiential or hands-on training, particularly for skills
- mini-lecture or brief didactic sessions presented by the resident.

Each of these methods can be enhanced by having fellow residents do some of the teaching or by combining the sessions with other disciplines, such as pharmacy or nursing. It is helpful to include direct observation of the resident–patient interaction to best determine what knowledge, skills or attitudes should be emphasized. Patients find this technique very acceptable and recognize this observation as physician contact time.

Creating the quality learning experience

Once you have assessed your own teaching style, determined the resident's preferred learning methods, and mutually agreed upon your intended outcomes, you can work to create a quality learning experience. The optimal learning climate matches a resident's ability with the level of teacher involvement (*see* Figure 4.1). Early in the training experience a resident may benefit from more dependent strategies to avoid anxiety, while a senior resident would benefit from more independent strategies to avoid frustration. By integrating the resident's current abilities, your teaching style and the desired goal, you will be ready to apply yourself to teaching situations that provide an optimal environment for learning.

Chapter 5

Dealing with Residents at Different Levels

Stanley M Kozakowski, MD

> **Key Points**
>
> - Learners are most successful when there is clear understanding about what is to be learned.
> - A mutually agreed focus for the teaching session may lead to a greater degree of satisfaction for both teacher and learner.
> - The educational focus may lead to specific teaching strategies for a given teaching session.
> - The care of patients is a complex task that can take years to master. Despite the general educational differences between residents at each level of training, significant variation in educational needs may exist between residents within the same postgraduate year of training.

In order to learn to drive a car, an individual must first learn the basic operations of the vehicle before going on the road. Initial simple rules are that 'stepping on the gas pedal makes the car go faster' and 'removing your foot from the gas pedal or stepping on the brake will slow the car.' The driver then begins to apply the basic principles within a variety of increasingly complex situations. With time and experience, he or she can learn to drive in a variety of conditions without much thought.[1] Likewise, physicians in training pass through different developmental stages. They progress from needing to think about everything they do to a state in which the care that they provide becomes 'automatic.'

Many preceptors believe that the learner simply needs to watch the preceptor and they will learn everything that is needed. Yet we would not simply say to a passenger, 'Observe me and you will learn everything that you need to know in order to drive.' However, learners are most successful when they are very clear about what it is that they are expected to learn. One strategy for achieving this goal is to understand the resident's needs based upon level of training and ability to implement a 'negotiated' plan for the teaching session. Few things are more frightening to a learner than not knowing what the teacher expects from them and not knowing the criteria upon which they will be judged. Creating a safe learning environment is the most respectful thing that a teacher can do for a learner!

The preceptor can identify the learner's needs by employing a number of different techniques. A good starting point is to recognize that most residents progress through a hierarchy of educational developmental needs. General needs are listed in Chapter 2. Box 5.1 lists examples of medical tasks for family practice residents by year of training. This list can be utilized as a guide for the preceptor, or when the resident is having difficulty articulating their needs for the session. The list can be shown to the resident and they can be asked 'Which of these would you be interested in using as a focus for today?' If the resident cannot or will not choose a particular task, then the preceptor can suggest one from the list. This process identifies individual competencies.

The preceptor should be aware that there may be significant differences between residents within the same year of training with regard to their educational needs. These differences will often be based upon the previous experiences of the resident (both medical school and their previous residency experiences).

Asking questions may help to identify the resident's educational needs. Examples of such questions include the following.

- 'What would make your experience a success today?'
- 'Tell me about your experience with patients with _____ so far in your training.'
- 'I am a more effective teacher if I have a specific focus for my teaching. We can talk about anything that comes up today, but I would like you to tell me what you are working on at this time.'
- 'Have you seen many normal _____ or abnormal _____ before?'

With an understanding of the resident's needs as a starting point, the preceptor should 'negotiate' an educational focus for the teaching session based upon the resident's needs and abilities and the resources of the preceptor (e.g. the number of residents in the session).

The preceptor should create and articulate a 'negotiated' strategy for the teaching session. This plan should outline the responsibilities of both the teacher and the resident. The plan can be based either upon an individual resident's needs or on the needs of the group of residents. Three examples are given below.

1 'Today we shall focus on creating full differential diagnoses for the patients that you see. After each patient's exam I want you to present to me a complete biopsychosocial differential diagnosis before we discuss any treatment plans. I will let you know if there is anything else that I can think of to put on the list.'
2 'Let us focus our teaching today on selecting cost-effective therapeutics. We shall talk about the cost of any medications that we may prescribe during today's session.'
3 'At the end of the session we will talk about all of your patients from the perspective of _____.'

Clearly articulated plans allow both the teacher and the learner to monitor the progress and the effectiveness of the teaching session.

Having a specific educational focus does not prevent the preceptor from addressing any issue. It merely provides a 'lens' for both teacher and learner and helps in creating a teaching strategy. The teacher should decide how much 'hands-on' experience they will allow for the learner if the patients are coming in to see the preceptor as the physician. Most residents desire as much 'hands-on' experience as possible.

Finally, the preceptor should provide closure at the end of the teaching session. Ask the resident what they learned today and if their educational needs were met. Help the resident to explore their 'next educational steps.'

Box 5.1 Hierarchy of Tasks by Year of Training

First-Year Tasks
- Identify the purpose(s) of the visit.
- Develop appropriate biopsychosocial hypotheses which apply to the presenting problem.
- Evaluate the presenting problem using a focused investigation, which will influence management decisions for this visit.
- Prioritize the probable and potential diagnoses to ensure that attention is given to the most likely, most serious and most readily treatable options.
- Present a provisional and working diagnosis to the patient.
- Develop a plan of action that attends to salient medical, ethical, spiritual, psychosocial, family, cultural and socio-economic issues.
- Arrange for follow-up of the current problem, which is consistent with the guidelines of current standards of care and/or meets the special needs of the patient.
- Conduct an interview, which should foster a nurturing doctor–patient relationship.
- Completely document the patient care encounter in the medical record in a concise and legible manner following a problem-oriented format and using the SOAP (Subjective, Objective, Assessment, Plan) notation.
- Update the biopsychosocial problem list and medication list at each visit.
- Bill the patient fairly and appropriately for services rendered (in accordance with their insurance option), referring those who need financial assistance to appropriate business office personnel.

Second-Year Tasks
- Implement the negotiated management plan.
- Inquire into and discuss sensitive issues that may impact on the execution of the negotiated management plan.
- If indicated, assist the patient in arranging for appropriate medical and ancillary referrals which seek to resolve specific issues in the diagnostic or management arena.
- Conduct an encounter which recognizes the primacy of patient needs and treats the patient as an appropriately equal healthcare partner.
- Conduct an interview in a manner consistent with the values of family medicine, utilizing appropriate verbal and non-verbal skills.
- Incorporate the principles and practices of health maintenance into each patient care encounter where appropriate.

- Review the biopsychosocial problem list at each visit and attend to appropriate longitudinal care issues.
- Conduct the visit in a time-efficient and professional manner.

Third-Year Tasks
- Work together with front-desk staff and nursing staff in a manner that fosters mutual respect and facilitates an effectively run office.
- Work together with partners, fellow family physicians and sub-specialists in a manner that fosters mutual respect and facilitates the effective handling of patient care issues.
- Work together with the rest of the healthcare team in a manner that fosters mutual respect and facilitates the effective handling of patient care issues.
- Complete the task of the defined patient care session so that all of the necessary tasks (including telephone messages, charting, administrative tasks and patient care) are accomplished in a timely, organized and professional manner.
- At each patient care encounter, present yourself, the practice and the specialty in a manner that will encourage the patient to select you, your practice and the specialty of family medicine in the future.
- Engage in continuing medical education activities, which are influenced by interest, deficiency and need.
- Engage in activities that will foster personal and professional growth (in mind, body, psyche and spirit) as a family physician.

Adapted from Bell HS, Kozakowski SM and Winter RO (1997) Competency-based education in family practice. *Fam Med.* **29:** 701–4.

Further Reading

Dreyfus SE and Dreyfus HL (1980) *A Five-Stage Model of the Mental Activities Involved in Directed Skill Acquisition.* Operations Research Center, University of California, Berkeley, CA.

Chapter 6

Providing Feedback: Goals and Objectives

Marian R Stuart, PhD

Key Points

- Feedback provides information for learners to help them to modify their behavior and reach their goals.
- Information that is based on direct observation and the observer's reactions (low levels of feedback) often prevents defensiveness in the resident.
- Shared goals and objectives provide a structure that facilitates learning, improves communications and simplifies the evaluation process.

Precepting medical residents in the office can be either an extremely positive or a frustrating experience depending on the degree of congruence between your expectations and those of the resident. Judicious use of feedback by both parties and the development of explicit goals and objectives for the rotation can do much to tilt the experience towards the positive pole.

Residents come to your office with a desire to gain clinical experience in the 'real world.' Constructing and discussing explicit goals and objectives for the rotation will focus your energies productively, inform the resident about what is expected and ease the evaluation process. Once the resident buys into the stated expectations, feedback can be used to ensure that the goals and objectives are met. Constructive feedback is experienced as a welcome gift that helps the resident to direct a course towards personal achievement.

Defining Terms

Let us be clear about a few definitions. *Feedback*, a term that Kurt Lewin originally adopted from rocket science in the 1940s, is information that lets people know where they are in relation to the goals towards which they are striving.[1] In practice, feedback is information that is shared with a learner about how a particular behavior is contributing to his or her achieving a desired goal. A *goal* is a global statement that describes the desired outcome of the rotation in terms of its effects on the learner. *Objectives* are specific statements that delineate the knowledge, skills and attitudes that must be acquired in order to achieve a goal.[2]

When residents are given the opportunity to work with a community physician for a period of weeks, the question becomes 'What changes in knowledge, skills or attitudes do we hope to see as a result of this experience?' The goal of the rotation might be to increase a resident's appreciation of the rewards of practicing medicine as well as their understanding of the complexity of managing a practice. In other words, the goal statement answers the question 'What is it that the resident will get from this rotation?' For each goal, several objectives should be developed that will detail the particular behaviors that would provide evidence of the achievement of this goal. The objectives fall into cognitive, psychomotor and affective domains – in other words, the particular knowledge, skills and attitudes to be attained.

Objectives need to be SMART – that is, **S**pecific, **M**easurable, **A**ttainable, **R**elevant and **T**ime-framed. Objectives answer the question 'By the end of the rotation, what specifically do I want the resident to now be able to do and/or feel?' *Specific* means who (in this case the resident) should be able to do or know what, how, when and under what circumstances. Objectives also need to be *measurable*. Knowledge components are *measurable* if the resident can describe, discuss, explain or analyze a particular phenomenon. Skills are *measurable* if they can be demonstrated and observed. Attitudes are inferred by the resident's willingness to engage in certain activities, promote certain practices or make particular commitments. Again the tool for measuring an affective objective is observation. *Measurable* also implies setting time expectations of how long a particular procedure or visit should take. *Attainable* means that it is reasonable to expect the learning to occur during the rotation. The objective should be *relevant* to the goal and achievable by the end of the rotation *(time-framed)*.

A discussion between you and the resident at the start of the rotation should clarify goals and objectives. This has the further benefit of assuring 'buy-in' and communicating clear expectations about what is to be learned, the resident's levels of responsibility and independence, and also the criteria for the summative evaluation of the resident.

Distinguishing Feedback from Evaluation

Whereas evaluation judges a performance against a standard or criteria and focuses on *how well* something was done, feedback provides information about *what* was done. Positive feedback provides information about observed behavior that leads towards the stated goal, whereas negative feedback provides information about behavior that is likely to deter residents from reaching their goals. Since human beings often become defensive when confronted with information which they anticipate might be unflattering or a challenge to their self-image, the lower the level of feedback, the easier it will be for the resident to hear and integrate the information. *Level 1 feedback* is by definition simply a description of the behavior that was observed, *level 2 feedback* provides information about the observer's feelings in relation to the behavior, and *level 3 feedback* provides information about the likely outcome if the behavior were to continue.[3] A useful way to remember the levels is as follows: level 1, *facts*; level 2, *feelings;* level 3, *forecasts*. There is no question that minimum resistance is encountered by offering feedback at levels 1 and 2.

Let us look at the following examples.

- **Level 1 feedback:** 'Just now while I was trying to give you some relevant history about the patient, you interrupted me to explain your reasoning.'
- **Level 2 feedback:** 'When you interrupted me, I felt frustrated and much less interested in spending time teaching you.'
- **Level 3 feedback:** 'If you continue to react this way, I'm afraid this rotation will be less valuable for you than it otherwise could be.'

Feedback should be specific rather than general, descriptive of actual behavior, directed toward modifiable conduct, occur as soon as possible after the observed behavior, and take into account the needs of both the preceptor and the resident.

1 Feedback should be timely. Provide feedback as close in time to the observed encounter as possible, in a neutral and concise manner.[3]
2 Feedback should be focused. It is most effective when it is focused on behavior and performance, and tied to specific actions. Merely saying 'great job' does not help the resident to focus on specific areas.[4]
3 Feedback should start with self-assessment. The preceptor should initially direct the resident to assess his or her skills and performance. For example, 'How did you think you did performing a knee exam?'
4 Feedback should be balanced. Let's consider the 'feedback sandwich.' Start with what the resident did well. Then suggest areas for improvement. Finally, reinforce what the resident did well. For example, 'You correctly diagnosed a breech presentation, but had difficulty performing Leopold maneuvers. However, it was important that you correctly identified a malpresentation.'
5 Feedback is a two-way process. Effective feedback requires candid communication between resident and preceptor. For example, 'What things could I be doing better to improve the quality of your experience in our clinic?'
6 Feedback should be concise and candid. Recognize and respect time considerations in a busy office practice. Be polite! Include brief, targeted 2- to 3-minute feedback sessions between patients. For example, 'I like the way you gently approached the frightened and agitated child, but if you have difficulty examining a squirming child, ask mother to hold him on her lap.'
7 Feedback should be future oriented. It should improve future skills and performance by involving the resident in developing a plan to enhance growth and development.[4] For example, 'It's obvious to me that you are interested in providing maternity care. As such, let's schedule additional time for you on the labor deck to enhance your skill base.'
8 Feedback must be honest and respectful. Feedback pearls include 'praise in public' and 'criticize constructively in private.' Feedback sandwiches are more easily digested!

Feedback given in liberal doses, both by preceptor to resident and also by resident to preceptor during the rotation, will result in achievement of the goals and objectives and a pleasant and productive learning experience for all concerned. Although all feedback is basically 'formative', encouraging improvement in performance, summative feedback given at the conclusion of the rotation that highlights specific observed strengths and weaknesses can also provide valuable information for the resident.

Box 6.1 Characteristics of Effective Feedback

- Formative
- Timely
- Given in appropriate location
- Specific
- Descriptive of actual behavior
- Modifiable behavior
- Tailored to resident
- Solicits learner's perceptions

Box 6.2 Example of Feedback

Setting: immediately after a difficult encounter with a depressed patient.

Preceptor: Let's go back to my office for a moment and discuss our encounter with Ms Jones *(appropriate location and timely)*. How do I feel about that encounter? *(solicits learner's perceptions)*

Resident: Well, I really thought I was doing well until I tried to ask about suicidal thoughts. Then I just didn't know how to ask.

Preceptor: I agree that you handled the encounter well – you were able to identify the pertinent positives and negatives of the patient's history to identify the presence of anhedonia and five other symptoms meeting the SMD–IV criteria for major depressive disorder. You then shared the diagnosis with the patient in understandable lay terms *(specific positives that are behaviorally linked)*.

Resident: Thanks. I have been really working on taking better psychiatric histories.

Preceptor: But I also agree you struggled a bit with asking about suicidality. Here is how I do it ... Does this make sense? Let's role play and have you ask about suicide *(formative, tailored to resident's need, and addresses specific, modifiable behaviors)*.

Resident: Thanks. I feel a lot better about taking a complete history of depression now. I can't wait to try this with a real patient!

References

1 Hanson PG (1975) Giving feedback: an interpersonal skill. In: JW Pfeiffer and JE Jones (eds) *The 1975 Annual Handbook for Group Facilitators*. University Associates, San Diego, CA.

2 Stuart MR and Krauser PS (2000) Using goals and objectives in community rotations. In: PM Paulman, JL Susman and CA Abboud (eds) *Precepting Medical Students in the Office*. Johns Hopkins University Press, Baltimore, MD, pp. 62–5 (this

material was originally developed by AE Rothermich, PhD at the Department of Family and Community Medicine, University of Utah, in 1978).

3 Ende J (1983) Feedback in clinical medical education. *JAMA.* **250:** 777–81.

4 American Academy of Family Physicians (2002) How to give feedback to learners. In: *The Advanced Life Supporting Obstetrics Instructor Manual.* AAFP, Leawood, KS.

Chapter 7

Performing an Evaluation

Kenneth G Reinert, MD

Key Points

- Evaluation is a dynamic educational process, the essence of which is resident quality improvement.
- The goals of an evaluation must be clearly defined and linked to outcomes.
- Evaluation serves to ensure that residents are meeting required standards.
- Evaluate against established standards and competencies.
- Evaluators should act on the results of the evaluations to improve resident performance.

Evaluation should be a positive educational process that contributes to professional development. An evaluation must be:

1 carefully considered
2 designed with clear goals and an established end point
3 linked to educational and healthcare outcomes.

The key is to evaluate against established standards and competencies.[1] Evaluation should address the resident's knowledge, skills, capabilities and attitudes for each area of the curriculum. Regulatory agencies have identified a series of core competencies that residents must master. Residency programs are required to ensure that resident physicians meet these competencies and standards. Evaluators must act on the results to correct deficiencies, improve performance and maximize the resident's potential. *Remember that evaluation is not an end in itself, but rather a process which ensures that residents meet established standards.[2] A residency program that produces an incompetent physician has betrayed its mission.[3] Accurate, valid and reliable evaluation is critical to residency training and resident quality improvement.*

Evaluation: Design Criteria and Characteristics

An evaluation must be carefully designed and adhere to established guidelines[3] (*see* Box 7.1).

Box 7.1 Characteristics of an Ideal Evaluation[1,4]

- Reliable, valid and accurate
- Inexpensive and easy to administer
- Paired with feedback
- Acceptable to the individual being rated
- Goals must be clearly defined and understood
- Employs measurable outcomes
- Includes both objective and subjective formats
- Includes quantitative and qualitative information
- Must address who is being evaluated (i.e. the level or year of training)
- Who will provide input? How will it be recorded?

Remember that evaluators must act on the results of the evaluation to enhance resident performance and development.

How Do We Evaluate?

Clearly, no single evaluation or assessment tool can provide the information required for objective judgment of performance as complex as the delivery of professional health services by a physician. Measurement of the candidate's knowledge base dominates current institutional and specialty examination systems. Evaluation must look beyond objective test scores and discern how residents integrate the competencies inherent to a successful medical practice.[5] A number of evaluation methods can be used to assess resident performance, including but not limited to oral examination, written tests, checklists, rating scales and standardized patient exercises.[6]

When to Evaluate

Evaluation is a dynamic process, the goal of which is resident quality improvement. The results should be shared with the resident in order to guide and enhance future performance. Early intervention can make a significant difference to a resident's performance.

Guidelines on When to Evaluate[1]

- Prior to each rotation – review written rotation goals, objectives and expectations.
- Mid-rotation – formative interim assessment used to provide feedback and/or plans for remediation.
- End of rotation – summative evaluation (i.e. a final grade which indicates whether or not standards have been met).

The Building Blocks of Evaluation

Fundamental components or building blocks that are essential for accurate resident evaluation include the following.[2]

1 **Formal review** of residency standards/competencies and summative evaluation procedures.
2 **Effective communication** between learner and evaluator formative feedback.
3 **Written documentation** that evaluations have been reviewed, understood and signed; plans to remediate, monitor and assist (written and signed).
4 **Due process:**
   - written standards reviewed and understood
   - well-defined and understood evaluation process
   - written plans to monitor and remediate reviewed and signed
   - defined consequences of failing to meet standards/competencies.

Remember that evaluation is necessary, valuable and follows established guidelines. Feedback is timely, focused and balanced.

However, in contrast to feedback, evaluation is a more formal judgment. It is an appraisal based on observations of how the resident met objectives and standards. Assessment results should be shared with the resident in order to correct deficiencies, provide remediation as needed, and enhance professional development. Evaluations must be documented, reviewed and signed by the resident.

Summary

Evaluation is a dynamic educational process designed to ensure that residents meet standards and reach the end point of their training program. The key is to evaluate against established standards. Evaluation and feedback allow residents to develop their skills and provide competent and effective healthcare.

References

1 *House Officer Evaluation: Enhancing Our Teaching Skills.* Madigon AMC Faculty Development Fellowship Series.
2 Short JP (1993) The importance of strong evaluation standards and procedures in training residents. *Acad Med.* **68:** 522–5.
3 www.acgme.org
4 Miller G (1990) The assessment of clinical skills/competence/performance. *Acad Med.* **65:** S63–7.
5 Snell L, Tallett S, Haist S *et al.* (2000) A review of the evaluation of clinical teaching: new perspectives and challenge. *Med Educ.* **34:** 862–70.
6 Morrison J (2003) ABC of learning and teaching in medicine. *BMJ.* **326:** 385–7.

Chapter 8

Teaching Challenging Residents

Jeffrey L Susman, MD

Key Points

- Recognize the role changes, personal challenges and environmental issues that foster difficulties in residency.
- Apply a four-dimensional approach to challenging learners.
  - Define the problem.
  - Divulge it (to colleagues and the learner).
  - Develop a plan of action.
  - Document and follow up.

Challenging residents, also known as 'problem learners' or 'learners in need', are a major source of frustration for full-time teachers and preceptors alike. The first suggestion of a problem may come from a patient, a colleague or the nursing staff, or it may arise from your own observations. In some instances, there may be a warning to 'watch Dr X like a hawk.' More commonly, a critical incident will arise unexpectedly – a resident is chronically late, a complaint filters to your front desk, or a medical assistant confides that she wonders how Dr X 'made it through medical school.' By understanding the challenges inherent in residency training and correctly defining the problem, a challenging situation can often be transformed into a rewarding one.

Presentation

Just like patients, our residents can be thought of as presenting with a chief complaint – for example, 'he is always late' or 'I can never trust his judgment.' Such 'symptoms' may accurately and transparently reflect the underlying problem, such as the resident who is 'all thumbs' who has had little experience of performing outpatient procedures. At other times the overt symptoms may reflect an underlying problem. Perhaps the resident who is late is trying to get their children off to school without much support from their partner. Occasionally, a critical incident will spark the problem, such as a resident who fails to show up for call, or who cannot be reached to deal with an emergency. Most likely it is a gradual dawning that 'there are problems' – a vaguer, less well-defined feeling that all is not well. Finally, the Residency Director may ask for assistance in helping a struggling resident with a specific area (e.g. procedural skills). The first step in any of these situations is to fully define the problem.

Defining the Problem

Initial assessment should include as many perspectives as possible, including those of nursing staff, patients and other colleagues. For example, a receptionist may notice how brusquely a resident treats staff when the attending is not present. Clarifying the accuracy and consistency of 'problems' can differentiate a one-time slip from more serious difficulties.

Moreover, a brief conversation may uncover a readily correctable source of difficulty. Perhaps a partner is concerned about a resident's knowledge base. If she has been used to having third-year residents on their rural experience, but all of a sudden a first-year resident comes to the office, solving the problem might be as simple as clarifying expectations. A call to the Program Director or the resident's advisor might also be helpful. Once a robust picture of the 'symptoms' has been painted, a tentative diagnosis can be made based on the following categories. Remember that many challenging learning situations are multi-factorial in nature.

- **System/environmental issues.** In some instances, the system or structure of the program or rotation may be at fault. Perhaps a general surgeon expects the resident to scrub in on cases at the same time as a partner expects the resident to make rounds. It is crucial to make sure that the expectations are realistic, that the resident is not in a double bind, and to clarify any challenges in the environment.
- **Teacher 'hypo-competency.'** In some instances, we have met the enemy and they are us! We may have forgotten to orient a resident at the start of the rotation and they don't know our expectations (*see* Chapter 4). Occasionally, there may be a mismatch of values or a mismatch of learner and teacher expectations, or differences in learning styles. For example, a very cognitively oriented learner may be unable to process information demonstrated by a preceptor during a procedure.
- **Knowledge-based issues.** These are common in residency. Of course, residents will be ignorant in many areas, which is why they are residents. Don't assume that knowledge-based deficits are across the board, or that the stellar resident doesn't have areas of weakness. Programs like Core Content or Home Study can provide programmed learning opportunities, as can learning assignments that are less formal (e.g. 'Why don't you read about the management of diabetic ketoacidosis, and we will discuss it tomorrow when we round on Mrs Smith.' Some residents have difficulty focusing in the free-form environment of the typical preceptor's office.
- **Psychomotor/procedural issues.** Even the most cognitively adept resident may lack psychomotor or procedural skills. It is not uncommon for a resident to have had less opportunity to perform procedures than they encounter in your practice.
- **Stress/psychosocial issues.** Given the stresses of residency, it is not surprising that depression, anxiety and other mental health issues arise. For example, learning that a resident has had a history of depression may clearly

explain his or her gradually deteriorating performance. Stress may provoke avoidance, a move towards substance use, or irrational hubris. As physicians we deal with such issues all the time in our patients – simply remaining alert for such possibilities will often allow us to make these diagnoses in our residents. Discussion with the Program Director and referral to appropriate resources (mental health or employee assistance) may be valuable.

- **Attitudinal/motivational issues.** Although fortunately uncommon, such difficulties are often the most provocative ones. Challenging situations may reflect other underlying problems, such as depression or difficulties due to family stress. Monikers such as 'lazy' or 'competitive' are not nearly as useful as clearly specifying problem behaviors – observable actions that cause challenges.

- **Cultural/linguistic issues.** With international medical graduates playing an increasing role in residencies, and US graduates continuing to be diverse, our own cultural and social biases may be a factor. A lack of eye contact and unwillingness to assume responsibility may reflect cultural norms with regard to how one treats a 'superior.' Adequate language skills for casual encounters may be stressed by the idiomatic communication of an unstructured outpatient rotation. In parallel with your initial evaluation of the 'presenting problem', including the gathering of corroborating data, you will also want to obtain the resident's perspective on this issue.

Divulging the Problem

One of the first steps in ascertaining the origin(s) of a challenging learning interaction will be to discuss the issue with the resident. Remember the value of an initial orientation (*see* Chapter 10) and the principles of constructive feedback (*see* Chapter 6). As with any feedback, soliciting the perspective of the learner can often be enlightening (*see* Box 8.1). It is surprising how often residents do have a sense of their shortcomings and opportunities for improvement.

Following the discussion of the problem, it is important to ensure communication with all parties involved in the resident's education. For example, you may have partners and staff who need to realize that your resident is trying to enhance his or her time management skills. If important deficiencies are found that merit longer-term follow-up, the preceptor should ensure that there is direct communication with the Residency Program Director or Coordinator.

Box 8.1 Divulging the Problem

Imagine this encounter when sitting down for coffee one morning after rounds.

Preceptor: 'So, Emily, how's the rotation going so far?'
Emily: 'Pretty good, I guess. I really enjoy the variety and responsibility of this rotation. I feel bad that I always have to leave right at 5:00 to pick up my daughter.'
Preceptor: 'Well, I'm glad you raised that issue. Dr Gruff was really frustrated when you took off yesterday without checking back on your new admission.'

Develop the Plan of Action

The plan of action will depend on the initial diagnosis of the problem (*see* Box 8.2). You will be able to handle many issues yourself, by carefully outlining a course of study, providing clear expectations with regard to performance, and assisting with further procedural skills instruction.

Just as with patient care, sometimes a trial of 'presumptive therapy' will help to clarify the diagnosis. For example, a resident who is chronically late may claim that they have extenuating domestic obligations. If problems persist, a more careful evaluation for mental health and substance use disorders may be in order. Challenging learners often present with multiple problems. A poor knowledge base and fundamental difficulties with language may have precipitated significant anxiety, which may in turn be associated with substance misuse and marital conflict. Only careful evaluation and follow-up will reveal the true cause and extent of any problem.

Box 8.2   Plans of Action for Selected Challenging Learners

- Systems/environment
  - Clarify responsibilities and expectations
  - Evaluate time constraints
  - Discuss goals of preceptorship with Program Director
- Teacher
  - Attend faculty development workshops
  - Use Preceptor Education Program materials
  - Attend STFM (Society of Teachers of Family Medicine), Residency Assistance Program or other educational conferences
  - Read other resources (see suggested readings)
- Knowledge
  - Suggest participation in a structured program such as Home Study or Core Content
  - Assign articles to read and discuss
  - Use Web resources (e.g. POEMs, Up-to-Date)
  - Model the use of learning resources
- Psychomotor/procedural
  - Suggest sessions at an educational skills laboratory
  - Provide opportunities to work with procedural specialists
  - Use supplemental CD-ROMs and videotapes
  - Facilitate participation in a course such as ALSO (Advanced Life Support in Obstetrics)
- Stress/psychosocial
  - Clarify priorities
  - Be alert for signs and symptoms that suggest drug use, depression or other psychosocial issues
  - Schedule regular time for unstructured, confidential follow-up
- Attitudinal/motivational
  - Establish a learning contract
  - Clarify resident's goals and perceived needs

- Ascertain specific barriers to learning
- Elicit student's help with other learners
- Cultural/linguistic
  - Get to know your resident's ethnic, religious and social background – maintain a non-judgmental attitude
  - Directly observe the resident's behavior and provide constructive feedback
  - Ascertain what resources might be available through the residency
  - Build on strengths

Document and Follow Up the Plan

One of the most important aspects of dealing with a challenging learner is appropriate documentation and follow-up. Documentation creates the legal basis for further action (even termination if necessary), a common understanding of the learner's needs among faculty and other preceptors, and an agreed plan for corrective action. Often the details of plans for remediation, particularly those involving serious shortcomings, will be the responsibility of a Program Director, chairperson or other medical school official, so good communication is essential. Most programs will have a due process procedure for more serious problems (such as gross negligence or harassment). Remember to notify relevant stakeholders locally, such as your hospital's legal department.

Plans for follow-up should be specific, actionable and clearly linked to an expected timeline. For example, if a resident is expected to expand his knowledge base, it is not enough to say 'read more.' A far better plan would be to specify that the resident is expected to read one Home Study monograph each week and be prepared to discuss its main points at noon each Monday. Such a plan is flexible (allowing the resident to learn in areas of his choosing) but specific enough to be 'actionable' (clear behaviors and a timeline are expected). Expressing expected changes in behavioral terms, such as 'I expect you to discuss each of your inpatients with the primary nurse, and to find out what the most important problem is from their point of view', is probably more likely to be successful than saying 'Make sure you work better with the nursing staff at the hospital.' A clear timeline, and in most cases a formal follow-up, will help to ensure that progress is monitored and deviations from expected behavior are discussed ('You are doing much better in making it to inpatient rounds on time, but you still get back to the office late after lunch'). Written documentation of each follow-up, mailed to the resident and the program, will ensure that your important observations are not lost. For most preceptors, ample assistance is available from the parent residency. Use this support regularly.

Summary

Challenging learners are often uncovered during preceptorial experiences. Seldom is the contact more direct and performance more closely observed than on a community preceptorship. When confronted with a challenging learner, the preceptor needs to define the problem and ensure that there is an adequate basis for decision making. A clear plan of action should be developed and appropriate communication and documentation should be established. Follow-up and feedback ensure that the 'loop' between the preceptor, trainee and program is closed.

Further Reading

Kahn NB (2000) Dealing with the problem learner. In: PM Paulman, JL Susman and CA Abboud (eds) *Precepting Medical Students in the Office.* Johns Hopkins University Press, Baltimore, MD.

Residency Services Committee, Association of Program Directors in Internal Medicine (1988) Stress and impairment during residency training: strategies for reduction, identification and management. *Ann Intern Med.* **109:** 154–61.

Steinert Y and Levitt C (1993) Working with the 'problem' resident: guidelines for definition and intervention. *Fam Med.* **25:** 627–32.

Yao DC and Wright SM (2001) The challenge of problem residents. *J Gen Intern Med.* **16:** 486–92.

Chapter 9

Teaching Ethics

Audrey A Paulman, MD

Key Points

- The community preceptor's office provides a unique training opportunity for ethics education for residents.
- Ethics training in the office should focus on issues of practical and immediate importance to the resident.
- All participants in the ethics education of residents have rights which must be respected.

Formal ethics education in medical school deals with issues that practicing physicians encounter, including confidentiality of patient information, end-of-life decisions, informed consent and assisted suicide. An informal ethics education occurs simultaneously as the physician in training observes and internalizes everything that is seen, heard or felt during the training program. As an educator of house staff, one must be aware of this shadow curriculum, which is taught all day, every day of the training program. Educators need to be comfortable addressing the new issues that present themselves as the students are transformed into house officers. Mentoring is a powerful educational tool. It should be used consciously and with attention to what is being taught.

Topics in ethics that are taught by the educator should be appropriate to the level of training and understanding of the house officer, and should be unique to that level of training.

Prescribing for Family Members

Preceptors need to address topics in ethics that are appropriate and unique to the house officer's level of training. Consider the following example.

A first-year house officer has a newly acquired ability to prescribe medications for family members. Laws governing prescribing behaviors vary from state to state, and acceptance of these behaviors varies from practitioner to practitioner. House officers observe attending behavior, whether it is appropriate or not. The attending physician should use this opportunity to help the house officer to understand the added responsibility and vulnerability of a physician who treats their own family members.

Dealing with Deception

There have been few studies of the use of deception by attending physicians. However, surveys indicate that house officers will occasionally use deception in order to change call, protect a patient, protect a fellow student or avoid performing a procedure. This behavior is not unique to house officers, but may be noticed in day-to-day activities with attendings and supervision of students. Keeping the level of training of the house officer in mind, the educator can seek ways to eliminate incentives to be deceptive. Again, the mentoring relationship should be used to help the house officer with these ethical decisions, both in his or her actions and in dealing with attending and students.

Claiming Responsibility for Mistakes

The house officer will choose to follow a mistake with either admission of responsibility, or denial. In addition, the house officer will have to address mistakes made by colleagues and attendings. The resident will question responsibility to the patient as well as a duty to confront errors. None of these choices are without significant risk, both within and outside the medical community. Making such choices for the first time may be a lonely process for a newly licensed house officer.

Addressing Problematic Behaviors

Problematic behaviors should be addressed. Behaviors such as showing disrespect for patients or taking medical short cuts are not acceptable. Preceptors have been shown to use non-verbal cues, such as posturing, facial expression or failing to respond, in order to show disapproval of house officers' problematic behaviors. Corrective actions for problematic behavior should be individualized, based upon the learner. However, the educator should be aware that a stressed physician in training may be unable to interpret subtle cues, and an immediate, direct, non-confrontational approach is more effective in helping the house officer to identify inappropriate actions.

Care of the patient is becoming more remote from the bedside. Computerized medical records, including on-screen radiographic images, nursing notes and vital signs, have taken the teaching away from the bedside and made it more remote from the patient. Conscious effort should be made to bring the teaching team closer to the patient, so that the resident learners can observe effective communication between the attending educator and the patient. This effective mentoring is important in helping the resident to develop a unique bedside style that will impact on future practice success and satisfaction.

Confidentiality

It is very important to discuss the confidentiality of patient information with any resident precepting in your office. The protection of patient information is a very practical application of ethical training in the office, and needs to be addressed explicitly with the resident at the start of the rotation. Besides being an ethical issue, patient confidentiality is now covered under federal law. Confidentiality is addressed further in Chapter 19.

Rights of Participants in the Ethics Education of Residents

The house officer has a right to:

- a good learning environment, with responsibilities matched to level of training and abilities
- be given feedback in a private and tactful manner
- decline to participate in procedures that conflict with their conscience
- admit to being unsure about his or her ability to participate in an activity due to personal skill or training
- not be treated in an abusive manner or harassed.

The educator has a right to:

- trust the house officer's word
- place his or her own responsibility to the patient above the house officer's need for an education
- tailor participation to the abilities of the house officer
- provide medical care conscientiously
- have a house officer ready to learn.

The patient has a right to:

- know that they are being seen by a physician in training
- give permission to be seen by a physician in training
- freedom from inappropriate relationships with caregivers
- receive the best and most appropriate care based upon their illness.

The Residency Training Program has a right to:

- receive honest feedback about a house officer's performance
- be confident that the house officer is in a reliable and ethical training site
- know that each person will be treated fairly without regard to race, gender, creed or ability
- provide support if the educator does not know how to handle a problematic learner.

Chapter 10

Orienting the Resident to Your Office

Dennis Baker, PhD, David Steele, PhD and Edward Shahady, MD

Key Points

- A structured orientation process is the foundation of a successful teaching and learning experience.
- A structured orientation consists of three components:
  - pre-arrival information provided to the resident
  - face-to-face discussion upon arrival
  - continuing orientation.
- Planning, conducting and reflecting are three phases of the orientation process.

It is common practice for residents entering the first year of their training program to undergo a formal orientation to the residency clinic and curriculum. These orientation programs usually consist of social, administrative and clinical components. However, when the resident does a rotation in a preceptor's office, a formal orientation is frequently absent. The resident shows up at the office, and the preceptor says 'Hi. I'm Dr Jones. Welcome to the practice. Follow me and we will start seeing some patients.' Wise residents can often deal with this situation because they have inquired about rotating in Dr Jones' office by talking to a peer resident who has already been there. A better alternative is a more formal and structured orientation that can greatly increase the effectiveness and satisfaction of the learning experience for the resident, as well as making the teaching process more enjoyable for the preceptor.

Why the Orientation is Important

A structured orientation is the foundation upon which a successful learning and teaching experience is built. The orientation:

- provides structure at the beginning of a learning experience
- clarifies how the teaching and patient care activities will be integrated, and thus makes both the teaching and the learning processes more efficient
- provides the opportunity to determine the resident's needs and strengths relative to his or her attitudes, knowledge and skills

- reduces the anxiety of the learner so that attention can be focused on learning
- provides an opportunity to establish a collaborative and positive relationship with the resident
- reduces the likelihood of preventable errors
- provides the opportunity for the preceptor to role model the educational value of an orientation for residents who will one day serve as preceptors themselves
- facilitates the opportunity for the resident to get off to a good start with staff and patients.

An Orientation has Three Components

Orientation, when it does occur, is frequently a 'one-shot deal.' However, the effectiveness of an orientation can be greatly enhanced by making it a multi-phase process that includes the following:

1 pre-arrival orientation (information given to the resident prior to their arrival at the office)
2 on-site orientation (face-to-face conversation with the preceptor upon arrival at the office)
3 continuing orientation (reinforcement of information from pre-orientation and on-site orientation).

Three Phases of the Orientation Process

The preceptor should:

1 **plan** all three phases of the orientation process
2 **conduct** the orientation, and then
3 **reflect** on how the process can possibly be improved for future residents he or she may teach.

Pre-Arrival Orientation Component

The pre-arrival orientation component helps the resident and preceptor to prepare for the face-to-face orientation. The pre-arrival orientation is a communication to the resident via e-mail or letter. This communication should convey enthusiasm for the resident coming to your office (e.g. 'My staff and I look forward to the time you will be working and learning in the office. We enjoy having residents and we have found that patients like them, too'). In addition to setting a positive tone, the communication should provide essential information such as the following:

- information about the staff (e.g. names, titles, roles)
- information about the practice (e.g. location, patient mix, number of patients, most frequent diseases and conditions seen, patient care guidelines followed)
- office routine (e.g. hours, scheduling procedures, chart data entry procedures, prescribing rules)

- information about the community (e.g. demographics, community resources for patients, other existing practices, hospital)
- expected arrival times and departure times, and expected dress
- information about how and when to contact you prior to the beginning of the rotation
- an inquiry concerning any special needs that the resident may have, such as a workspace, or access to a computer and printer.

The preceptor should also send a copy of this communication and accompanying information to the residency director so that he or she is fully informed and can be confident that the resident will be spending time with a preceptor who is organized and provides a good learning environment.

The content of the pre-arrival orientation communication and accompanying information should lay a foundation for a face-to-face meeting with the resident. The communication should ask the resident to make a list of procedures (skills) and diseases/conditions (knowledge) about which they would like to learn more. This will help the resident to clarify his or her learning needs, and it takes the task beyond the 'I'll be thinking about it' stage.

On-Site Orientation Component

You are now ready to conduct the face-to-face orientation with a focus on:

- creating a collaborative relationship
- helping the resident to identify their learning needs
- setting expectations for feedback.

The pre-arrival communication has established a foundation for this. Thirty minutes is usually sufficient for this meeting.

We often hear the statement 'You never get a second chance to make a good first impression.' An enthusiastic warm greeting, good eye contact and some small talk will help to create a relaxed and humanistic atmosphere. Sharing some information about your own family and interests will set the tone for the resident to do likewise. An important next step is to set the stage for the beginning of a collaborative teaching and learning experience. The essence of a collaborative teaching/learning environment is that the teacher and learner work together as a team and learn from each other. This might be expressed as follows: 'I look forward to this teaching opportunity. I have the experience of being in practice for ten years and I try to keep up with practice guidelines on the diseases seen in my practice, but I also know that in your residency clinic you are constantly exposed to cutting-edge information, so I look forward to learning from you, too.'

Assess the resident's learning needs by asking them to discuss the skill and knowledge areas that they want to work on during the rotation. The key is to discuss them in some depth and to clarify which of these competencies the resident will be able to work on in the practice and which of them are likely to be accomplished. Suppose that the resident identified joint injections as a procedure that they wanted to work on. The preceptor can conduct a needs assessment and simultaneously facilitate the resident's skill in self-assessment by asking specific questions such as the following.

- How many joint injections have you done?
- What types of patients did you do them on?
- How did it go when you did them?
- What parts of doing the procedure were easy? What parts were difficult?

It may take some time for the resident to become comfortable expressing what is difficult or easy, or how they feel about the quality of their performance, but as the preceptor and resident get to know each other and trust is developed, these exchanges will become much easier.

Ask similar questions about the resident's knowledge area. The resident might indicate that they want to gain more knowledge of the management of elderly patients with type 2 diabetes. Similar questions can be asked.

- Have you seen many elderly patients with this condition?
- What was your approach when working with these patients in the residency clinic?

An honest and realistic self-assessment of learning needs expressed by the resident is very much linked to the atmosphere that you establish in the face-to-face orientation and the tone set by the pre-arrival communications. In order to accurately self-assess and let the preceptor know about his or her needs, the resident must feel that the learning environment is safe and non-judgmental.

In addition to exploring knowledge and skills it is important to address attitudes. Attitudes impact on the acquisition of skills and knowledge and also on how knowledge and skills are used. It is important to allow the resident to express her attitudes with regard to certain types of patients and the associated behaviors involved in their care. For example, you may have a number of patients for whom you are providing smoking cessation programs. Knowing the resident's attitude towards patients who smoke and towards efforts to help those patients is invaluable for you as a teacher. Questions such as 'How do you feel about patients who smoke and are unable to quit?' or 'What has been your experience with helping patients to quit smoking?' will give you important information about the resident's attitude.

We have stated that establishing a collaborative atmosphere and working with the resident to identify their learning needs are two important components of the face-to-face orientation. These two components naturally set the stage for a discussion on feedback and how and when it will be given (feedback is addressed in Chapter 6). Asking the resident about past experiences of feedback will reveal attitudes towards this matter that you should take into account as you work with the resident to formulate feedback strategies.

The preceptor should also give the resident the opportunity to ask questions about the pre-arrival materials. In addition, make it clear to the resident how the coordination of teaching and patient care activities will be conducted. Allowing the resident to share their thoughts on this matter will make the resident more invested in the orientation process and will also demonstrate your sincerity about being collaborative.

Introducing the resident to your office and nursing staff should be an extension of the on-site orientation. Staff acceptance of the resident is critical for a successful learning experience. Sometimes residents have a negative feeling towards staff resulting from their hospital experiences. The relationship that you display with your staff serves as a model to the resident and will be an important part of what he or she learns in the office. Let the resident know how important the staff are to your success.

Continuing Orientation Component

Everything that the resident needs to know in order to be successfully integrated into your office practice cannot be covered in the pre-arrival and initial face-to-face orientation phases of the orientation process. Therefore the first week of the rotation should be thought of as a continuing orientation process. At the end of the week, time should be scheduled for you to sit down with the resident to review orientation topics as needed and to answer any questions that the resident may have generated during the week. This component of the orientation process provides the preceptor with the ideal opportunity to address anything that might be developing into a problem (e.g. arriving late, improper charting, inappropriate interactions with staff).

Reflecting on the Complete Orientation Process

Planning, conducting and reflecting are 'phases' of the orientation process. The effectiveness of teaching is enhanced by reflection or 'thinking back.' Reflection is a process that is easily neglected. It is important to reflect both on things that went well and on things that could be improved relative to all three components (pre-arrival, face-to-face and continuing orientation) of the orientation. It is important to make some notes as each component occurs. Then making reflective notes on the entire process, perhaps early in the second week of the rotation while memories are still fresh, will be helpful. Feedback from the resident and staff can also be incorporated into these notes. Sharing your notes and thoughts with a colleague or staff member can also be valuable. This reflection process is the key to making orientation the foundation of an effective learning experience for residents.

Further Reading

Alguire PC, DeWitt DE, Pinsky LE and Ferenchick GS (2001) *Teaching in Your Office.* American College of Physicians, Philadelphia, PA.

Baker SD and Gray-Starner L (1992) Intern orientation: obstacle or opportunity? *J Am Osteopath Assoc.* **92:** 501–6.

Steele DJ (2000) Orienting medical students. In: PM Paulman, JL Susman and CA Abboud (eds) *Precepting Medical Students in the Office.* Johns Hopkins University Press, Baltimore, MD.

Westberg J and Jason H (1993) *Collaborative Clinical Education.* Springer Publishing Company, New York.

Whitman NA and Schwenk TL (1984) *Preceptors as Teachers.* University of Utah School of Medicine, Salt Lake City, UT.

Section II

The Teacher and the Learning Environment

Chapter 11

Involving Your Office Staff in Teaching

Dale R Agner, MD

Key Points

- Learning the roles and functions of staff members will enhance the resident's experience.
- Many staff members have much to offer (e.g. coder, quality manager, nurse educator).
- Introduction of staff and discussion of expectations for both the resident and staff members facilitate the resident's learning.

The accumulation of knowledge does not necessarily impart wisdom.

(Dale R Agner)

The practitioner's office is the key environment where the resident learns to translate medical facts acquired in books, lectures and wards into the art of medicine in the outpatient realm. Indeed, understanding the biochemical process of diabetes does not mean that the resident will be able to teach the patient how to modify their diet or to convince them of the need to start medical therapy. Since the physician is a part of the healthcare delivery team, understanding the roles and functions of the team members can facilitate a more thorough understanding of the practice and application of the medical principles that the resident is learning. The intention is to provide ideas or resources within the office or business practice for which office staff may provide adjunctive perception to the resident.

Interpersonal Skills: How the Resident Relates to Staff and Patients

Bedside manner and being a team player are key skills for which the office staff can help to provide feedback, model or teach. Spending lunchtime, a couple of hours or a couple of days with the following people or functions can hone or develop invaluable interpersonal skills for the resident.

Each office usually has a person who functions as a patient advocate or an ombudsman for patient complaints. Spending time with the person designated the 'Patient Advocate' can provide valuable insights. This may be accomplished by observation, discussion of past cases, or participation in an active complaint.

Allowing the resident to research a patient complaint can provide valuable insights for him or her. In addition, it could assist the office by allowing 'fresh eyes' to evaluate a process (this could also be performed in a quality review process, such as researching how a critical pathological report became 'misplaced').

The office staff also develop opinions and receive feedback from patients about the resident. Asking the staff to provide feedback to you can be quite helpful (*see* Box 11.1). The clinic/rotation preceptor may wish to review these comments before the resident receives them (e.g. to ensure that the comments are appropriate or to provide a context for comments that the resident may not understand).

Box 11.1 Feedback by Staff

It can be quite helpful to ask the staff to provide feedback to you on the following:

- ability to work with others
- ability to relate to patients
- ability to manage an appointment efficiently (how efficiently the resident may have seen a patient independently)
- ability to provide clear and understandable instructions or medical explanations to patients (a staff member is often the person to whom a patient will confide if they did not understand an instruction or medical explanation).

Business and Practice Management Skills: How the Office Works

The coding, billing and office administrators have skills to teach which are invaluable to the resident. The person who provides coding oversight has much practical knowledge to impart, including information about the common pitfalls encountered while coding. The resident may also review his records with the coder in order to gain additional insights. In addition, reviewing charts for Medicare compliance can be instructive.

Staff involved with quality improvement also have much to offer, as they teach the systems that will evaluate the physician in the future.[1]

Learning how to operate and maintain the equipment within the office can also be instructive.

Processes Within the Office

Many offices have someone designated for patient education or management of specific diseases (e.g. diabetes, asthma, dysplasia). The resident could have his or her notes/record reviewed with a nurse educator regarding a disease with well-known clinical practice guidelines (e.g. asthma, diabetes or cardiovascular disease). The resident could also observe, follow or take on specific projects with the person(s) responsible for healthcare integration within the office setting.

Specific projects could include obtaining pharmacy data for patients diagnosed with persistent asthma, to ensure compliance with controller therapy. Residents could review diabetic records for evidence of compliance with evaluation and management guidelines.

Preparing the Resident and the Staff for Precepting Within the Office

Lastly, it is also important to discuss with the staff the resident's role within the office setting during the rotation.[2] If the staff perceive the resident as someone who slows down the clinic, the resident will miss learning opportunities. Preparing the resident to be a learner from the staff, and preparing the staff by assuring them that they have something to offer the resident, can help the learning experience for all.

Conclusion

The office staff can facilitate the process of becoming a skillful artisan in the practice of medicine.

Office staff can be key players in providing information to the preceptor about the resident's interpersonal skills and bedside manner. Office staff interactions and the lessons that they can provide are crucial to the education of residents.

References

1 Houry D and Shockley LW (2001) Evaluation of a residency program's experience with a one-week emergency medicine resident rotation at a medical liability insurance company. *Acad Emerg Med.* **8:** 765–7.
2 Moser S, Callaway P and Kellerman R (2002) Involving the office staff in teaching medical students. *Fam Med.* **34:** 565–6.

Chapter 12

Integrating Practice Management into the Preceptorship

Kaye Carstens, MD

Key Points

- Practice management knowledge is essential for a successful practice.
- The preceptor's office provides unique practice management learning opportunities for residents.
- Specific time slots must be allocated regularly for effective learning of practice management.
- Real-life experiences facilitate practice management learning.

A practice management curriculum should include but not be limited to the areas of personal finance, office and personnel management, business planning, electronic medical records, managed care, alternative practice models, professional liability and risk management.

Early in their training, residents have little interest in practice management, but towards the end of their training, practice management issues become more important. Physicians who are looking for employment suddenly realize that business skills are a necessity in today's medical economic environment.

Most physicians' offices are very busy and leave little time for the preceptor and the resident to focus on the business aspects of medicine. For this reason, it is best to schedule a specific time each week so that practice management is not overlooked. Emphasize to the resident that all practice business information is confidential and is best left at the office.

Personnel Management

It is key to give the resident permission to ask questions about the business aspects of medicine, because some residents feel that this information should not be discussed. Office efficiency and atmosphere depend on how employees function and perform their job duties. Residents need to understand that each employee in the practice fulfills a specific function and requires direction to accomplish it. A specific job description for each employee is key to efficient office operation. In addition, appropriate and thorough job descriptions depersonalize issues that may arise, such as discrimination. The resident needs to have an understanding of the business aspects of the following positions: practice managers, front-desk personnel, book-keepers, laboratory staff, X-ray technicians and floor assistants.

Residents should spend time with the nurse or medical assistants in order to understand their role in the process of care, such as reviewing the next day's patient list, looking for orders to be carried out before seeing the physician, making sure that instruments are ready, taking phone messages, securing information for the physician, and ensuring that the rooms are ready.

Practice Partnership or Corporation

Physician practice can be either a partnership or a corporation. The resident should study these business models in order to fully understand the differences between them, as well as the advantages and disadvantages of each model. Sharing personal experiences can be helpful.

Malpractice Insurance

Issues of resident coverage are dealt with in Chapter 19. A resident transitioning into practice needs information on different types of malpractice insurance. The office manager would be a good resource for reviewing the type of policy held by the preceptor. Key concepts for the resident are the limitations and coverage of each type of policy, including the following:

- claims made
- occurrence
- tail policies.

Basic Accounting Principles

Every business needs a system to reflect its financial status. This system provides information about revenues, expenses and profits. It will also reflect what the business owns (its assets) and what it owes (its liabilities), and what the business is worth (capital, net worth or equity). The income statement and the balance sheet present a picture of the clinic's financial statement. The income statement includes revenues minus expenses that equal income. Income minus the physician's salary is recorded on the balance sheet that includes assets, liabilities and capital (net worth). The resident must understand that cash flow is a month-to-month projection about adequate cash to operate your practice and meet your personal living expenses. If the practice is new and just expanding, it may need financial backing until appropriate cash flow is achieved. Financial institutions are willing to make loans to young physicians, as they are considered to be a good risk, but they will need to have a comprehensive practice business plan and cash-flow budget. Credit-worthiness is influenced by how much is to be borrowed, proposed use of the money, repayment plans, the practice outlook and the character of the borrower.

Two methods of accounting are cash and accrual. When cash accounting is used, the revenues and expenses are posted to the period in which the money is actually received or spent. Under the accrual method, the revenues and expenses are posted to the period in which they are earned or incurred. Most physicians' practices use the cash basis. This method is simpler and requires less work, but it doesn't provide as precise a financial picture as the accrual method. The resident should learn basic accounting principles, including the following:

- ensuring maintenance of good accounting control
- yearly audit of the practice's books by the accountant
- coverage of staff members under a fidelity bond
- reviewing bills when paid
- number and account for encounter forms
- daily balance of day-sheets
- alertness for variance in petty cash
- understanding the 'cash cycle.'

Planning Beyond Residency

Retirement plans are common among many businesses. To attract good office personnel and partners to the practice, retirement plans need to be included. The Employee Retirement Income Security Act governs pension and retirement plans. Many retirement plans are available, and the type may vary from practice to practice. Many clinic practices have defined contribution plans that include profit sharing and money purchase pension plans. Whatever type of retirement plan you as a physician have, this is a good opportunity to give an in-depth education to the resident. Explain the various components of the plan, such as how much the employee and employer contribute, the time required before the employee is fully vested, and at what age withdrawals can be made for retirement. The resident should also understand the basic types of personal insurance, including health, life and disability coverage, and the types of policies available.

Conclusion

The resident has an excellent opportunity to experience hands-on learning of practice management via immersion in the preceptor's office. A systematic approach to business education and practice management will enhance the resident's education in the preceptor's office.

Further Reading and Useful Websites

Valancy J (1999/2000) *The Complete Practice Management Seminar. General Accounting 5.1–5.8. Personnel 7.1–7.4.* Jack Valancy Consulting; www.valancy.com/pdf/tcintro.

Kalogredis V and Burke MR (1997) Working out your buy-in. *FPM.* **4(9)**.

Kalogredis V and Burke MR (1997) Building a solid employment agreement with a small group. *FPM.* **4(4)**.

Arnow FM and Xakellis GC (2001) Making your balance sheet work for you. *FPM.* **8(6)**; www.aafp.org/fmp (10 June 2003).

Chapter 13

Dealing with Regulatory Bodies, Acronyms and Resident Hours

Jeffrey D Harrison, MD

Key Points

- There are multiple regulatory bodies governing graduate medical education.
- Documentation of appropriate supervision will cover most regulatory concerns.
- There are now rules that restrict the number of hours that residents can work.

There are multiple regulatory bodies governing residency education. Their individual requirements and areas of oversight are not necessarily congruent, and an understanding of each of their individual functions and goals is needed in order to maintain appropriate compliance.

The major regulatory body for all graduate medical education (GME) in this country is the Accreditation Council for Graduate Medical Education (ACGME). Within the ACGME each specialty has a Residency Review Committee (RRC) that sets the educational requirements for that specialty. The Center for Medicare and Medicaid Services (CMS), formerly known as HCFA, sets forth the regulatory guidelines for residents who are dealing with Medicare patients. The Joint Commission for the Accreditation of Healthcare Organizations (JCAHO) has recently increased the oversight of resident activities and privileges within the hospital and hospital-managed clinics. Finally, individual hospital medical staff may have specific regulatory guidelines concerning resident activities. The following sections will expand on each of these regulatory bodies and outline the general requirements that they have set out.

Accreditation Council for Graduate Medical Education (ACGME)

ACGME is a private professional organization responsible for the accreditation of nearly 7,800 residency education programs in 110 specialty and sub-specialty areas.

Any institution, whether it is a hospital, university or foundation, that wishes to sponsor graduate education programs must comply with the Institutional Requirements of the ACGME. Educational oversight of each training program is to be provided by an institutional Graduate Medical Education Committee. The duty of this committee is to see that the institutional requirements are being implemented and met by the individual programs. The ACGME's major area of focus currently involves resident work hours and resident competency.

The resident work-hour rules came into effect on 1 July 2003, and encompass all graduate educational programs regardless of specialty. The current work-hour guidelines are as follows.

- Residents cannot be on duty for more than 80 hours per week averaged over a 4-week period.
- Residents cannot evaluate any new patients after being on duty for more than 24 hours. A 6-hour period for transfer of patient care and education is allowed, but the resident must be off duty after 30 hours.
- Home call will count towards the 80-hour limit if the resident is required to return to the hospital.
- Residents must have one day in seven away from the program, averaged over a 4-week period.
- In-house call may not occur more often than every third night averaged over a 4-week period.

The ACGME has developed a set of six core competencies, which are outlined in Chapter 15.

In the office setting, the ACGME regulations that will require preceptor awareness include total work hours per week and post-call duties by the resident. It is also important for the preceptor to remember that they will be expected to provide some evaluation of the resident with regard to the six core competencies.

Residency Review Committee (RRC)

Each medical specialty has an RRC that accredits each individual program, as well as setting the specific program requirements for their specialty. The RRCs function under the direction of the ACGME. Membership of the RRC consists of representatives of the Specialty Boards, the Specialty Academies and the American Medical Association.

Specific program requirements regulated by the RRCs include the following:

- duration and scope of training
- institutional organization
- faculty qualifications and responsibilities
- facilities
- educational program
- evaluation process.

Faculty qualifications and responsibilities, the educational program and the evaluation process are the three areas that will impact on precepting in the office. Preceptors are expected to possess the appropriate certifications by their specialty boards and to have a strong interest in residency education. All major components of the educational program should have written goals and objectives, as well as a methodology for teaching the material. Finally, a system must be in place not only for evaluating the resident's performance, but also for evaluating the preceptor and the educational experience.

In the office setting, the RRC regulations that will require preceptor awareness include the expectation that preceptors are interested in teaching. They should also be aware that there exist written goals and objectives with regard to the experience, and they can expect to receive a copy of these. The preceptor should also realize that in addition to evaluating the resident's performance, both the preceptor and the experience must be evaluated by the resident.

Center for Medicare and Medicaid Services (CMS)

The CMS is concerned with the billing and documentation practices as they relate to its beneficiaries. It provides funding to graduate medical education programs through Part A of Medicare. That funding supports residents' salary and education. Providers (preceptors) bill Medicare through Part B. The CMS is not willing to pay the resident through Part A and then again through Part B. The expectation of the CMS is that the billing provider (the preceptor) will provide the service for which they are generating a bill. The CMS is willing to have residents involved in the care of its beneficiaries. However, it is not willing to pay the resident twice (via Parts A and B) for providing a service.

The basic tenet for preceptors to follow when dealing with CMS beneficiaries is that the teaching physician (preceptor) will document their involvement in the key portion of the encounter. For the typical E&M (evaluation and management) visit, the key portions are the history, exam and medical decision making. For procedural-based visits, it is essentially documenting presence for the entire encounter. Resident documentation is allowable and should be referred to by the preceptor. However, independent documentation of involvement by the preceptor is needed if a bill is to be generated. Lack of preceptor documentation in CMS beneficiaries where a bill is generated is considered by the CMS to constitute fraud or abuse.

In the office setting, the CMS regulations mandate that the preceptor (the teaching physician) documents his or her involvement and physical presence for any encounter in which a bill is generated for a CMS beneficiary. If no preceptor documentation is possible, a bill should not be generated.

Joint Commission for the Accreditation of Healthcare Organizations (JCAHO)

The JCAHO is an independent, not-for-profit organization that accredits and evaluates over 15,000 healthcare organizations in this country. Although this organization does not deal directly with residency education issues, it is concerned with standards and quality of healthcare.

For those practices that are hospital-based or accredited JCAHO ambulatory centers, written policies need to be in place relating to what activities a resident may perform. Specifically, organizations should delineate what residents at various levels of training are allowed to do and how that decision is made.

In the office that is JCAHO accredited, there will need to be a written policy as to what residents are allowed to do and how that decision is made.

Hospitals/Group Practices

Preceptors should be cognizant that their hospitals and group practices may have guidelines and regulations with regard to residents.

Useful Websites

ACGME; www.acgme.org
CMS; www.cms.gov
JCAHO; www.jcaho.org

Chapter 14

Documenting Supervision

Eric Skye, MD

Key Points

- Supervision of residents in the outpatient setting is regulated by the Center for Medicare and Medicaid Services.
- The teaching physicians must ensure that the care provided by the resident physician is appropriate.
- The scope of practice of residents is dictated by the scope of practice of the precepting physician.

Supervision of the resident physician in the outpatient clinical setting has undergone significant changes over the last 10 years. Historically, the level of supervision and the resident's scope of practice were largely dependent on the supervising physician's assessment of the skills and needs of the resident. The establishment of the *Supervising Physicians in the Teaching Settings* policy[1] by the Health Care Financing Administration (now the Center for Medicare and Medicaid Services or CMS) brought government regulation to the forefront of resident supervision standards. For any physician or practice caring for Medicare beneficiaries and submitting billing to Medicare for those services, this policy essentially sets the standard for the level of supervision that must be provided to the resident physician, and this will therefore be the focus of this chapter.

The key principle in supervising resident care is that the teaching physician must ensure that the medical care provided is appropriate. In an attempt to ensure this overseeing of a resident physician's care, the CMS requires that the teaching physician either personally performs the service or is 'physically present during the critical or key portions of the service that a resident performs.' The 'critical or key portion' of a service is determined by the teaching physician, and will vary depending on the patient and the required medical care. For example, a patient presenting with an exacerbation of asthma might have the assessment of their respiratory status and determination of a treatment plan identified as the critical portion of their care. Another patient presenting with the same condition might require, as the key portion of their care, appropriate counseling on the use of their medications. It is the teaching physician's responsibility to define and be present for these 'critical or key' components. A caveat to this guideline occurs during visits that are billed on the basis of time. By billing by time you have defined the key component of this visit as the time spent with the patient. You can only bill on the basis of time if the teaching physician was actually present for that specified amount of time.

The documentation of medical care provided in the teaching setting allows a resident's note to be counted so long as the teaching physician personally adds a statement indicating that they were present during the key portions of the service or includes any participation they had in performing that service. Examples of acceptable statements as provided by the CMS include the following.

- *I saw the patient with the resident and agree with the resident's findings and plan.*
- *I saw and evaluated the patient. I reviewed the resident's note and agree, except that the picture is more consistent with pericarditis than with myocardial ischemia. Will begin NSAIDs.*

The teaching physician may always provide their own documentation of patient care and the services that they provided. The guidelines allow for a combination of the resident's and teaching physician's notes, which minimizes the need to repeat documentation.

The scope of practice of a resident physician is limited to that of the teaching physician, as the final responsibility for appropriate care is that of the teaching physician. This includes the performance of various procedures in the office and in hospital. The supervision of procedures requires not only that the teaching physician be present during the 'critical or key portion' of the procedure, but also that they are always immediately available to return to the procedure. For example, a patient presenting for a skin biopsy might be counseled and 'prepped' by the resident, and the teaching physician could confirm the area to be biopsied and assist in the performance of the biopsy. If you have previously determined that the resident has appropriate skills in skin suturing, you could allow the resident to suture the biopsy site without your physical presence, but you must be available to immediately return if your presence is required. Your documentation of this service could include the resident's note with a statement by you indicating your presence and immediate availability, such as '*I was present and participated in the key portions of this procedure and I was immediately available for the entire procedure.*'

An exception to these procedural guidelines occurs with any procedure that takes less than 5 minutes to complete. For these 'minor' procedures the teaching physician is required to observe the entire procedure, and should note their presence in their documentation.

Many family practice and other primary care residency programs qualify for an exception to the guidelines discussed above. The purpose of this exception is to allow residents to provide care to a group of established continuity patients. The requirements for this exception are designed to allow the resident's primary training clinic to qualify, and would not usually be fulfilled by the practicing physician teaching residents in their office. Therefore these will not be discussed here. Further information about this exception should be found in the resident's training program or by reviewing the CMS policy.[1]

The supervision guidelines discussed above are specific to Medicare patients, but provide an evolving standard for the supervision of resident physicians. The key issue in providing supervision for the resident is recognizing that, as the teaching physician, you are responsible for ensuring that the care which is provided is appropriate. Regardless of the payor or billing requirements, when teaching residents your personal involvement in any medical care should always be sufficient to ensure that there is appropriate care, and it should be adequately documented.

Reference

1 Centers for Medicare and Medicaid Services (2002) Fee schedule for physicians' services. In: *Carriers Manual Part 3*; www.cms.hhs.gov/transmittals/downloads/ R1781B3.pdf.asp (accessed 17 April 2006).

Chapter 15

Addressing ACGME Competencies

Karla Hemesath, PhD *and Jeffrey A Stearns,* MD

Key Points

- Residents must achieve proficiency in competencies described by the Accreditation Council of Graduate Medical Education (ACGME).
- Office teaching strategies can help residents become proficient in these competencies.

Significant changes are occurring in graduate medical education, and one aspect of change is the introduction of instruction in and evaluation of resident performance in six key competency areas, namely patient care, medical knowledge, professionalism, interpersonal and communication skills, practice-based learning and improvement, and systems-based practice. This switch to competency-based instruction, learning and evaluation was prompted in large part by the regulatory body of graduate medical education, the Accreditation Council of Graduate Medical Education (ACGME): 'The residency program must require its residents to obtain competencies in these areas to the level expected of a new practitioner.'[1]

As preceptors, programs will be relying on you to address aspects of competencies in your day-to-day teaching and also while you observe and assess resident performance. The purposes of this chapter are as follows:

1 to provide an overview of each competency
2 to identify practice behaviors and skills that fall into each category
3 to review some teaching tools that will help you to address these areas in your work with residents
4 to review some practical tools that you can use to assess resident performance in these areas.

Competency Overview

Although some of the competencies, such as patient care, medical knowledge, professionalism and interpersonal skills, are not new to graduate medical education and are relatively easy to define, the other two, namely practice-based learning and improvement, and systems-based practice, are less familiar to residents and preceptors. We have provided brief descriptions below, and Box 15.1 lists the specific skills required for each competency.

Patient Care

In essence, the patient care competency encompasses 'what the resident does'[2] in his or her day-to-day activities to diagnose and treat illness. Essential components of the patient care competency include history taking, physical examination skills, diagnostic ability, procedural competence, and appropriate prescription of therapeutic interventions.

Medical Knowledge

This competency represents 'what the resident knows'[2] and his or her ability to apply it to clinical situations. The key areas include ability to apply relevant knowledge, understanding and application of relevant basic science information to clinical situations, and analytic thinking to solve clinical problems.

Professionalism

Professionalism is a broad area, but it can be defined globally as 'how the resident acts.'[2] Each preceptor has their own definition of what professionalism is and what they expect of residents rotating in their office. Central areas in professionalism include professional responsibility, reliability, respect for patients and patient diversity, an ethical foundation and decision-making skills.

Interpersonal and Communication Skills

The interpersonal and communication competency is broadly defined as 'how the resident interacts with others.'[2] Central skills in this competency include ability to develop and maintain ethical relationships with patients and colleagues, appropriate clinical communication and documentation, case presentation skills, and the ability to work as a team member.

Practice-Based Learning and Improvement

Basically this competency highlights 'how the resident learns about their practice and does quality improvement.'[2] The essential components of this competency include reading, accessing, evaluating and appropriately using scientific evidence in their provision of care, accepting and utilizing feedback from attendings and colleagues, and identifying areas for improvement both in day-to-day practice patterns and from patient data.

Systems-Based Practice

A simple definition of systems-based practice is 'how the resident works within the system.'[2] Key areas include consultation, care coordination, accessing ancillary services, practice management, and billing and coding (*see* Box 15.1 for a summary and overview of each competency).

Box 15.1 ACGME Core Competencies[2]

Patient Care: What the Resident Does
Residents are expected to provide patient care that is compassionate, appropriate and effective for the promotion of health, prevention of illness and treatment of disease, and at the end of life.

- Gather accurate, essential information from all sources, including medical interviews, physical examinations, medical records and diagnostic/therapeutic procedures.
- Make informed recommendations about preventive, diagnostic and therapeutic options and interventions that are based on clinical judgment, scientific evidence and patient preference.
- Develop, negotiate and implement effective patient management plans and integration of patient care.
- Perform competently the diagnostic and therapeutic procedures considered essential to the practice of internal medicine.

Medical Knowledge: What the Resident Knows
Residents are expected to demonstrate knowledge of established and evolving biomedical, clinical and social sciences, and the application of their knowledge to patient care and the education of others.

- Apply an open-minded, analytical approach to the acquisition of new knowledge.
- Access and critically evaluate current medical information and scientific evidence.
- Develop clinically applicable knowledge of the basic and clinical sciences that underlie the practice of internal medicine.
- Apply this knowledge to clinical problem solving, clinical decision making and critical thinking.

Practice-Based Learning and Improvement: How the Resident Improves
Residents are expected to be able to use scientific evidence and methods to investigate, evaluate and improve patient care practices.

- Identify areas for improvement and implement strategies to enhance knowledge, skills, attitudes and processes of care.
- Analyze and evaluate practice experiences and implement strategies to continually improve the quality of patient care.
- Develop and maintain a willingness to learn from errors and use errors to improve the system or processes of care.
- Use information technology or other available methodologies to access and manage information, support patient care decisions and enhance both patient and physician education.

Interpersonal and Communication Skills: How the Resident Interacts With Others

Residents are expected to demonstrate interpersonal and communication skills that enable them to establish and maintain professional relationships with patients, families and other members of the healthcare team.

- Provide effective and professional consultation to other physicians and healthcare professionals and sustain therapeutic and ethically sound professional relationships with patients, their families and colleagues.
- Use effective listening, nonverbal cues, questioning and narrative skills to communicate with patients and families.
- Interact with consultants in a respectful, appropriate manner.
- Maintain comprehensive, timely and legible medical records.

Professionalism: How the Resident Acts

Residents are expected to demonstrate behaviors that reflect a commitment to continuous professional development, ethical practice, an understanding and sensitivity to diversity and a responsible attitude towards their patients, their profession and society.

- Demonstrate respect, compassion, integrity and altruism in relationships with patients, families and colleagues.
- Demonstrate sensitivity and responsiveness to the gender, age, culture, religion, sexual preference, socio-economic status, beliefs, behaviors and disabilities of patients and professional colleagues.
- Adhere to principles of confidentiality, scientific/academic integrity and informed consent.
- Recognize and identify deficiencies in peer performance.

Systems-Based Practice: How the Resident Works Within the System

Residents are expected to demonstrate both an understanding of the contexts and systems in which healthcare is provided, and the ability to apply this knowledge to improve and optimize healthcare.

- Understand, access and utilize the resources, providers and systems necessary to provide optimal care.
- Understand the limitations and opportunities inherent in various practice types and delivery systems, and develop strategies to optimize care for the individual patient.
- Apply evidence-based, cost-conscious strategies to prevention, diagnosis and disease management.
- Collaborate with other members of the healthcare team to assist patients in dealing effectively with complex systems and to improve systematic processes of care.

Teaching Strategies

Don't let the terminology and scope of the competencies overwhelm you. As an office preceptor your primary responsibilities with regard to the competencies are fairly straightforward.

1 Become aware of the competencies and understand the elements of each that apply to your specialty.
2 Pick one or two relevant and practical aspects of each that you can build into your regular resident teaching routine.
3 Discuss with your resident the competency areas to which they believe they need most exposure.
4 Observe and assess the resident's progress in each area so that you can briefly address it in the end-of-rotation evaluation.

In other words, find practical, concrete examples and applications of each competency in your day-to-day practice. These simple and concrete behaviors will reinforce the key points and will influence resident learning and practice.

Teaching Ideas

Some specific teaching tools that you can use to incorporate competency-specific teaching include pre-rotation briefing, topic review, case discussion, chart review and directed reading. If the program you work with sends out rotation goals and objectives, start with these. Briefly reviewing these with your resident will help you both to identify areas that can be addressed during the rotation. It is likely that you address multiple areas of each competency in your day-to-day work, but it is important to highlight this for the resident. Clearly communicate to the resident your expectations about their role in the care of your patients, what knowledge you expect them to gain during your rotation, the professional expectations that you have of them, and the manner in which you prefer them to interact with you, your partners, staff and patients.

Evaluation Assistance

Ideally, if you have addressed the ACGME competencies with the resident and have incorporated competency-specific points in your teaching routine, evaluation of the resident's performance will be simple. Keep in mind the following questions.

1 Does the resident understand the concept?
2 Are they able to demonstrate it?
3 Do they understand why it is necessary?

The American Board of Internal Medicine (ABIM) offers some specific tools that have been designed for preceptor and attending use, namely the mini-clinical evaluation exercise (mini-CEX) and the 'competency card.'[3] Both the mini-CEX and the competency card are small, pocket-sized checklists that allow you to keep notes and record resident performance. They are fairly simple in design and offer methods for keeping track of resident-specific data. The CEX is encounter-specific and gives the rater an opportunity to evaluate the resident's skill on multiple portions of a patient encounter. The competency card lists each competency and provides prompts that can help the faculty to identify aspects of the competencies and record information about a resident's performance. Samples are available from the ABIM website.[4] Your best resource for resident evaluation is the evaluation form provided by the residency. It will identify the criteria by which you evaluate the resident's performance, and this is your best roadmap for giving feedback to the resident during the rotation and for evaluation at the end of the rotation. These forms will probably increasingly utilize competency terminology, and it will be important to understand the specific behaviors, knowledge and skills that they are asking you to evaluate.

Summary

The ACGME competencies represent a shift in focus and outcome for residency education. Although this shift is important, it is not as complicated as it looks. As a preceptor, being aware of the competencies and the behaviors relevant to your practice is your best preparation for resident teaching and evaluation. Once you recognize common aspects of the competencies in your day-to-day work, you will be able to draw connections and actively teach residents about these issues in your care of patients.

References

1 Accreditation Council of Graduate Medical Education Outcome Project. Approved September 28, 1999. *General Competencies: Minimum Program Requirements Language*; www.ACGME.org/outcome/comp/compmin.asp (accessed 2 July 2003).
2 Tomasa L, Lebenshon P, Gordon P *et al.* (2003) *A Checklist of Core Competencies for First-Year Residents. STFM Conference on Patients and Families.* Kiawah Island, SC.
3 Norcini JJ, Blank LL, Arnold GK and Kimball HR (1995) The mini-CEX (Clinical Evaluation Exercise): a preliminary investigation. *Ann Intern Med.* **123**: 795–9.
4 www.abim.org/pubs/default.htm

Chapter 16

Working with the Residency Program and Site Visits

Richard Fruehling, MD

> **Key Points**
>
> - A good working relationship between the residency program and community physician preceptors will enhance the education of residents.
> - Residency programs can provide critical support to the community preceptor for the education of residents.
> - An explicit plan for teaching residents in the office will enhance the resident's education.

The decision by a physician to become a resident preceptor is made from many different directions. A recent graduate may want to maintain contact with a program they have come to enjoy and respect. A recent retiree may view involvement as a way to continue an enjoyable, lifelong career, and hope to pass on their experiences to a new group of physicians.

Most preceptors are motivated by an interest in maintaining and improving their own skills and helping the medical novitiate to begin that same lifelong process. Whatever vector brings the physician to that decision, being a resident preceptor is like everything else in life – it's not as simple as it seems!

Usually the preceptor involvement begins with a contact from the Residency Director of a program. That contact may be initiated by either party, but the subsequent process is the same. The director will supply an orientation. The level of orientation will be based on the size of the program and the needs of the preceptor.

The most important part of the orientation is exposure to and an understanding of the goals and objectives for the particular resident rotation. Every residency program will have these documents. The 'Gs & Os' help both the preceptor and the resident to maximize the learning opportunities. After some experience with the 'Gs & Os', the preceptor's feedback to the residency program will be appreciated!

Most preceptors have not previously been exposed to adult learning theory. The exposure to different learning styles of individual residents can be an eye-opener. Some guidance from the Residency Director of the residency program can be expected, but a good basic textbook on learning theory can ease the stress that the preceptor may experience (this is also discussed in Chapter 4).

One of the better teaching guides is *The One Minute Preceptor: Five Micro-Skills for Clinical Teaching.*[1]

Many new preceptors are surprised and confused by the residents' curricula. The educational plan of all residencies is based on sound educational theory and adapted to the local medical environment. Residents may be required to spend time in their 'continuity clinics.' The time varies from specialty to specialty. Frequently the new preceptor is not aware of this requirement, and trying to arrange a rotation schedule so that appropriate patients are available for the resident can be a frustrating exercise. It is the responsibility of the resident director and the individual resident to keep the preceptor informed of the resident's 'non-rotation' clinic times.

The governing body for residency education is the ACGME (*see* Chapter 13), which designates Residency Review Committees (RRCs) for each specialty. The RRCs set the program requirements and review each program to ensure that those requirements are being fulfilled. As part of the RRC's review process, a site inspection visit is required. The frequency of these visits is determined by the RRC based on the previous history of the individual program. This process is not dissimilar to the hospital reviews by the Joint Commission for the Accreditation of Healthcare Organizations (JCAHO). At the time of the site visit, the RRC wants the following documentation 'available for perusal by the site visitor on the day of the visit':

1 written goals and objectives for all curricular components and evidence of their distribution
2 resident contract/agreement
3 documentation of resident eligibility for appointment to a residency for graduates of non-LCME (Liason Committee for Medical Education) schools
4 evidence of evaluation of residents, faculty, the program and graduates
5 the full conference schedule with names of presenters, topics, and when presented
6 evidence of resident documentation of experiences and procedures
7 written supervisory policies of the residency
8 letters of agreement with ambulatory facilities
9 formal grievance procedure.

The involvement of the individual preceptor with this process is usually quite limited. The Residency Director and staff will, however, be stressed! Usually the RRC reviewer wants to meet for a short visit with some of the resident preceptors. This is a way for the reviewer to determine that the program has properly involved the preceptor with orientation, goals and objectives, and evaluation criteria. This process is part of the evaluation of the program, not of the preceptor. The preceptor will receive a request for involvement in the site visit process several months before the actual visit. The Program Director can be expected to review the possible questions that may arise during the RRC visit.

Reference

1 Neher JO, Gordon KC, Meyer B and Stevens N (1992) A five-step 'microskills' model of clinical teaching. *J Am Board Fam Pract.* **5**: 419–24.

Chapter 17

Preparing the Community and Practice for the Resident

Jeffrey W Hill, MD

Key Points

- Issues which need to be addressed for the integration of the resident into the preceptor's practice include the following:
  - housing
  - assimilation into the community.
- Helping the resident to assimilate into practice and the community will enhance the educational experience for faculty and residents.

Community Issues

Housing

If the preceptor site requires the resident to be away from home, there are unique considerations. Preceptors may or may not provide housing. Flexibility in housing needs is key. Appropriate, comfortable accommodation is important for the resident to feel welcome in the community. Resident physicians may come alone or may possibly bring a spouse or partner and perhaps children as well, so housing arrangements have to be flexible. If education will be a continuous feature in the medical practice, consider purchasing a home or identifying permanent rental property. It is important for the residents and their families to feel comfortable in the community. This comfort facilitates good working relationships and allows their assimilation into the community. The medical staff need to discuss the financial implications of housing and education for resident rotations. Items to consider and discuss include the following:

1 basic housing needs
2 utility bills (including responsibility for excessive use of utilities or phone)
3 Internet access and acceptable use
4 special needs due to disability of the resident.

Community Integration

An important aspect of the preceptorship is exposure of the resident to community activities and resources. Introducing the resident and possibly their family to community leaders is an appropriate step in this process and allows the resident to assimilate well into the community. Participating in community events and being 'welcomed' are important parts of making the resident feel at ease, and allow the community to potentially recruit the resident into the practice in the future. Publicizing the resident's arrival in the community newspaper and having a short biographical sketch available help the community to welcome the resident and understand the educational mission of the practice. This publicity may help patients to feel more comfortable seeing the resident. This publicity conveys the message that education is important and that residents will be learning 'real-world' medicine.

Maps and event schedules for the local community are helpful. Residents are highly visible in small communities and should be briefed on unique community cultures.

Food, Laundry, Transportation and Paging

- The resident who is away from home will often eat in the cafeteria of the hospital, and arrangements need to be made for this.
- Sometimes laundry is available for scrubs. Orientation on the rules for this is helpful.
- Transportation to off-site rotations is usually the responsibility of the resident.
- A system for local paging or telephone needs to be secured.

Medical Integration

Staff Training

Involving the staff is an important part of resident education. The educational faculty should review the goals and objectives of the resident's education, and relate the experience level and needs of the resident to areas where he or she needs further instruction. Office staff provide an important part of the evaluation of the resident's experience. They also have an excellent feel for the complexity of the patient population of the office, and are able to lend a helping hand and direct the resident with potentially difficult patients. Scheduling patients with complex problems for the resident should be avoided initially. Staff can provide insight into patients' social and family issues and community resources. As the resident's experience level increases, more complex issues can be dealt with, especially if there are important learning issues to be gained from such encounters. The staff are also invaluable for obtaining feedback – both positive and negative – from the patients, and also for evaluating the resident's ability to interact with the patient both cognitively and technically (e.g. residents performing gynecological exams and pap smears). In addition, the staff can expedite the resident's efficiency by teaching him or her common protocols of the office.

Providing Patients for the Resident

Patient scheduling is dependent on the level of training of the resident. Junior residents typically can see four to six patients per half-day, whereas senior residents can see up to 12 patients per half-day. The resident can be eased into the practice by scheduling patients with complaint-specific or simplistic problems until he or she is comfortable with both office and protocol. Patient flow can be monitored and adjusted according to the comfort level of the resident, which eases faculty supervision. Patient flow can be accommodated if the residents have their own space in which to work that is complete with reference materials, standard office forms and a procedure manual. There are several ways to schedule residents. The least preferable method is to have the resident see the attending physician's schedule of patients first and report key findings, followed by the resident and physician in tandem returning to the room for completion of the encounter. A more efficient method is to have a modified wave system in which several patients are scheduled at the same time, allowing faculty and residents to see patients simultaneously. The attending physician's pace is usually faster, which allows staffing of a simultaneous patient when a faculty patient encounter is finished. A third method is to let the resident have their own schedule of patients, making contact with the attending physician only at times when there is a need for clarification of patients' problems, the teaching of a procedure or discussion of a disease entity with which the resident is not familiar. It is important for the supervising physician to make contact with the patients whom the resident treats in order to maintain the doctor–patient relationship as well as facilitating billing issues.

Call Schedule and Time Away

New residency work rules require resident physicians to work not more than an 80-hour week, with at least one full day off per week, and residents must have an uninterrupted 10-hour interval between patients following a night on call, as noted in Chapter 13. This includes moonlighting activities. Flexibility of the resident's schedule is key here. A typical working week could include the resident being in the office for four full days with two nights on call. This schedule would also allow ample time for opportunities to participate in acute care cases as well as night call without violating the work-hour rule. Knowing their working schedule in advance allows the resident time to be part of the community and participate in local events, and to meet their family commitments.

Conclusion

Ensuring that living accommodation is comfortable, publicizing the educational mission of the office with resident education, and allowing the resident to gain

Table 17.1 Sample Working Week

Sun	Mon	Tue	Wed	Thu	Fri	Sat
Off	Rounds + Office	Rounds + Office	Rounds + Office	Rounds + Office	Office	Office
Off	Office	Office Call	Off	Office	Office Call	Off

experience and confidence are important keys to maintaining efficiency, patient flow, and satisfaction with the educational process both for the attending physician and for the resident. By meeting with the resident on a frequent basis, objectives can be identified and met, deficiencies identified and corrected or remediated, and the resident allowed to feel part of the practice. The needs of the community as well as those of the attending physician can thus be maintained.

Chapter 18

Collaborating with Local Hospitals

Michael R Gloor, FACHE

> **Key Points**
> - A thorough hospital orientation will enhance the resident's educational experience and improve patient safety.
> - Patients will often consider residents to be full medical staff. Therefore the resident should be familiar with the hospital bylaws and regulations.
> - It is imperative for both resident education and patient safety that the resident is familiar with the information technology and medical record systems of the hospital.

Most hospitals, regardless of their size, are training sites for a wide variety of technicians and clinicians. The addition of medical residents to the mix is usually easily accommodated. However, the nature of their training usually requires a far more thorough orientation to a veritable labyrinth of programs and services. Having the physician preceptor intercede or assist in this orientation is not only important for your charge to have a good learning experience, but also for the safety of your patients.

For most physicians, interacting with an acute care facility has become second nature – not so for the medical resident. Given that the residents will be visiting institutions of varying sizes, the level of orientation necessary may vary dramatically. Larger institutions will probably have a formal orientation. Calling the medical director's office may give you a one-time/one-stop opportunity. Intermediate-sized institutions may require 'delivering' your charge to a variety of departments in order to complete the orientation. With smaller institutions you may sometimes be required to orient the resident based upon your own knowledge of hospital operating procedures. For any of these cases, the intention of this chapter is to provide you with a general list of issues, protocols and policies that should be covered in an orientation to specific departments of the hospital. Try to overcome the urge for both resident and preceptor to 'hit the road running.' Do so in the interest of patient safety, the well-being of the resident and the enhancement of the resident's educational experience.

Departmental Orientation

Start the orientation with a tour, and if at all possible do it yourself. Show the resident where to park, and show them the obligatory doctors' lounge, where they can hang their coat, where they can grab a cup of coffee, etc. Although many hospitals are willing to provide the orientation tour, walking the halls and becoming familiar with the layout under the wing of their preceptor is usually far more beneficial for the resident. Don't forget the social connection. Introduce them to nursing staff (whose knowledge and skills you trust) and radiologists (who may be willing to spend extra time tutoring them on imaging, etc.). Don't underestimate the importance of this first step. First impressions are the most lasting ones.

Administration/Medical Staff Office

Make this your first stop for two reasons.

1 Depending upon the size of the institution, they may be able to handle the entire orientation.
2 They will be able to pave the way and open the doors for the rest of the orientation.

Because patients within the hospital often perceive residents as full medical staff members, expect this department also to inform the resident of bylaws and some general rules and regulations for practitioners, as well as the hospital confidentiality policy. Should the resident be invited to a 'moonlight' within a department, such as the emergency room, he or she will be required to undergo the hospital's credentialing processes prior to such activities. A stop at these offices will also give the resident access to keys, keypad codes, parking tags and an occasional freebie, such as a meal ticket.

Information Technology

A quick orientation to information technology (information systems) has become an imperative in almost all hospitals. The resident will need to understand the technology available, as it can vary widely from hospital to hospital. Examples of this can include assessing patient information online, entering orders, rounds reports, Internet access to medical information, etc. Passwords and some orientation will be required to utilize these important tools.

Health Information (Medical Records)

The health information department maintains the patient record and other vitally important patient data. There are a variety of topics related to orientation that can be important to residents, such as how to access dictation equipment to dictate patient reports, medical record completion requirements, and privacy guidelines on how to handle patient information in accordance with various state and federal privacy regulations. For their own protection, residents may also be requested to sign confidentiality agreements that outline specific expectations related to privacy and security. This is also a good time to introduce the resident to the utilization review process that is used to determine the appropriateness of admissions and continued stays and medical necessity requirements by third-party payors. This is an important stop, but it can also be overwhelming, as the amount of orientation that can be provided here is almost limitless. Good intentions not withstanding, try to rescue your resident from this stop after a reasonable amount of time.

Laboratory/Diagnostic Imaging

There are a number of clinical departments with which the medical resident may interact, including, but not limited to, the cardiopulmonary, therapy, dietary and pharmacy departments. The laboratory and diagnostic imaging departments are selected in this chapter only because the frequency of interaction with these two departments far outweighs that with most other clinical departments. The exception, of course, would be pharmacy. However, the pharmacists or the nurses will usually find their way to the medical resident to provide a degree of orientation and assistance pertaining to administration of medications, formularies, etc.

The key issues that can be addressed in orientation to these two key clinical departments are concerned not only with scope of services, which is again dependent upon the size of the institution, but also with the hours during which these services are available, which can also vary widely. Even departments that are open 24/7 quite frequently cannot provide all tests on a 24/7 basis. Some laboratory tests may be performed on a referral basis with a reference laboratory. The procedure for ordering tests and the method of receiving results as well as the time frames behind results should be fully explained. The availability of a pathologist or radiologist and the method for obtaining a consultation will help to identify the support and resources available to the resident. Most laboratories have critical value reporting and special standard operating procedures, such as automated differentials with a manual differential reflexed by certain triggers. Pertinent forms, test catalogs and collection guides are helpful aids for medical residents who will be ordering tests. An awareness of the availability of blood and blood products, as well as the estimated time for product preparation, may be essential for some medical residents. Wait times for some imaging modalities seem to be an inevitability, and the orientation can point out the modalities where this is most likely to occur. Again, some of these points can be extrapolated to other important clinical departments. Your perspective on many of these points will add a 'real-world' component to the orientation. As was stated earlier, don't forget the personal touch of introducing the resident to the pathologist(s) and radiologist(s). This improves the chances of engaging them in mentoring roles.

Surgery

Unless the resident is a surgical resident, it is doubtful that orientation to surgery needs to be undertaken during their first days with you as preceptor. Inevitably the day will come when the resident will be exposed to or rotated through the surgical department. Expect them, regardless of their training, to be tested on and re-oriented to sterile technique.

Most surgical departments have their own orientation process and will take charge of the resident, whether it's a lecture on the importance of scheduled start times or an explanation of the pecking order in locker assignments. The staff of surgery are usually better prepared to do the orientation than you as preceptor. Trust their judgment.

Emergency Services

Orientation to the ER is usually very limited unless this is the resident's training site. Unless the resident will see your personal patients when they present to the ER, a brief walk through by the preceptor will suffice. Anything more thorough is best left to the head of the department.

Educational Services

The educational services departments of hospitals provide many resources to assist medical residents. While each differs in its scope of service, most of these departments instruct, coordinate or have registration information on basic and advanced life support courses, as well as a broad range of other educational activities. Residents may attend accredited CME activities provided by hospitals, along with local physicians, and may also utilize the hospital library, which provides access to computers and the Internet, medical textbooks and journals, and assistance with research. A visit or even a phone call can provide direction to the resident on how to access the Internet, be placed on mailing lists for programs, etc.

   Near the beginning of this chapter it was noted that active practitioners consider many of the interactions listed previously to be second nature. However, try to empathize with the medical resident who may be overwhelmed when faced with the reality of being a stranger in a very technical and procedurally driven institution. Review the lists above and add your own perspective to the issues or topics, especially as they relate to the size of the institution involved. Remember that almost all components of the orientation format have been put in place over a period of time for reasons that relate to the safety of both the patient and the resident. Time spent orienting to the hospital will be time well spent.

Chapter 19

Addressing Liability Issues

Amy L Longo, JD and Alan Lembitz, MD

Key Points

The following legal objectives should be met when participating in the clinical education of medical residents:

- providing quality care and treatment for your patients
- providing residents with sufficient clinical education to evaluate fairly their abilities to meet the objectives of the clinical rotation
- avoiding exposure to liability for acts or omissions throughout the educational experience.

The following is a discussion of actions that you can take to make the clinical educational experience beneficial to your patients, the resident and yourself.

Orientation

From a legal standpoint, before residents engage in clinical education they should be provided with an orientation to the office. This orientation should include the following areas.

1 **Introduction to office staff.** If the resident is to function safely in the office, he or she should be introduced to the staff and understand each staff member's responsibilities. The resident should know which staff members he or she is expected to interact with during the clinical experience.
2 **Review of office policies and procedures.** If the office has written policies and procedures, the resident should be given the opportunity to review and clarify these before participating in clinical activities in the office.
3 **Infection control.** Although the resident should be well trained in infection control prior to assignment to a clinical rotation, he or she should be instructed in the infection control policies and procedures of the office.
4 **Use of equipment.** The resident should be aware of any equipment used in the regular course of the office practice, and should demonstrate proficiency before using it.

Patient Rights

Informed Consent

Respect for the patient and sensitivity to the concerns of the patient eliminate many potential legal problems. Emphasizing the patient's right to consent to or refuse treatment is basic to patient care. The legal elements of informed consent include the following.

- Explanation of the proposed treatment, the inherent risks and benefits of treatment and the alternatives to treatment.
- Providing adequate time, under the circumstances, for the patient to ask questions.
- Giving the patient the option of withdrawing consent at any time.
- When considering whether the patient is giving *voluntary consent*, the following should be considered:
  - Does the patient have the ability to understand your explanation?
  - Is there any outside pressure from other individuals causing the patient to agree to the treatment?

The person providing the treatment should obtain consent from the patient. If a resident is treating a patient, they should tell the patient that they are a resident. Patients have the right to refuse treatment. This includes the right to refuse treatment by a resident. If the physician plans to have a resident participate in the patient's care, he or she should inform the patient of the resident's role. Generally patients do not object to having residents participate in their care. However, if a patient does not want a resident to participate in their care, the patient's request should be respected.

Confidentiality

Patients have the right to keep their medical information private. State and federal laws protect this privacy right. Under the federal Health Insurance Portability Act of 1996 (HIPAA), the office of a physician is required to adopt privacy protection for patient information. The office is required to have policies in place addressing confidentiality of patient information. When a resident has a clinical rotation in a doctor's office, the resident must be educated about the Office Privacy Policy and must sign a statement stating that they understand the policy and agree to comply with it.

In general terms, the resident should be aware that a patient's medical record should be discussed only in a private setting, and that no patient information should be revealed without the patient's permission.

Malpractice

The potential lawsuit creates grave concern for all physicians. For the teaching physician, the concern is not only for the physician's own acts but also for the proper supervision of residents.

The elements of malpractice include the following:

1 duty owed to the patient
2 breach of the duty to the patient by act or omission by failure to meet the standard of care
3 injury to the patient proximately caused by the breach of duty.

When a physician is supervising residents, he or she must be aware of the resident's clinical abilities and be available to the resident to the extent necessary for the resident to perform the delegated duties in a manner consistent with the standard of care applicable to the physician. Therefore the physician should be aware of the educational level and clinical experience of the resident, before delegating patient care and treatment to him or her. This awareness should come from communicating with the educational program and the resident, and from the physician's direct instruction and observation of the resident. Further information on orienting residents at different levels can be found in Chapter 5.

Malpractice Insurance

It is always advisable to review malpractice insurance coverage in order to be certain that coverage is provided for supervision of medical residents. Residency programs should have malpractice coverage for residents.

Resident Legal Rights

Evaluation of Performance

Residents have the right to expect a fair evaluation of clinical performance. The residency program should provide guidance to the physician who is supervising a resident's clinical rotation concerning the areas of resident performance that are to be evaluated and the form of evaluation.

Nondiscrimination

Residents have the right to clinical education in an environment that is free from discrimination on the grounds of gender, race, national origin, age or disability. A resident who is in the physician's office should:

1   be aware that discrimination, including harassment, will not be tolerated
2   be told who to contact if the resident believes that he or she is being subjected to discrimination.

Chapter 20

Using Educational Resources

Michael Horn, MD

Key Points

- Preceptors can look to a number of organizations for continuing medical education credits in order to improve both their teaching skills and their skills as physicians.
- The American Medical Association and the Joint Commission for the Accreditation of Healthcare Organizations both provide educational materials on the topic of patient safety.
- Preceptors can also find societies and publications that discuss issues such as quality improvement, end-of-life issues, documentation and coding guidelines.

Medicine has been and will remain in a state of flux and accelerated change not seen in a century. Those responsible for preparing new physicians need to prepare themselves and their trainees for this time of transition. There are a variety of support services and products available for community preceptors.

Continuing Medical Education

Continuing medical education (CME) for preceptors can be divided into two distinct categories. The first concerns preparation and skills related to teaching and education in more general terms, and the second is the traditional CME by which one maintains skills and current competency.

With regard to the first, there are two primary resources available to the preceptor in addition to the chapters in this book that deal with the topic. The first of these is the Society of Teachers of Family Medicine (STFM).[1] On their website can be found *Office-Based Teacher*, which is an archive of articles addressing topics of interest to community preceptors, sponsoring organizations, students and residents. The STFM also has an online bookstore and sponsors national seminars of interest. Through the bookstore, modules for the Preceptor Education Project (PEP) are also available. These can be used either for independent self-learning or within the context of locally provided seminars.

Among the seminars available through the STFM is the Faculty Development Series. This set of five seminars ranges from the basics of instructional planning and design to taped critiques of the preceptor's presentation style, research design, and even managerial and administrative skills. It is intended for community preceptors as well as for those in academic settings who wish to pursue a formal course of study to improve their skills.

Preceptors can also access support materials through local Area Health Education Centers (AHECs) or their affiliated academic institutions. Generally the preceptor will be aware of the local AHEC and its point of contact. However, there is also the National AHEC Organization (NAO),[2] which serves as a clearinghouse. There are multiple links from its website to other AHECs. Many of these local AHECs have been in existence for some years and have developed a wealth of resources.

The second main category of CME is the traditional one aimed at maintaining and improving physician skills. Working with students and residents is always an exciting and challenging adventure in which both student and teacher learn. To keep pace with emerging young physicians, preceptors will need to keep their own knowledge base strong and up to date. CME is now widely available in a variety of formats, including Web-based instruction. Many hospitals are accredited to provide CME, and State Medical Societies in cooperation with the Accreditation Council for Continuing Medical Education (ACCME) can accredit organizations that are seeking to provide their own CME. The American Academy of Family Physicians (AAFP)[3] can also provide CME credit for specific programs that meet format and content requirements. The AAFP should be contacted prior to the presentation in order for it to be properly documented.

Emerging Issues

Of the changes that are being seen in medicine and medical practice, one element which is unlikely to change for some time yet is the emphasis on improved quality and patient safety. From the expansive, even exaggerated claims of the initial report by the Institute of Medicine (IoM), 'To Err is Human', in 2000 to its follow-up, 'Crossing the Quality Chasm', and a host of other reports and articles, this issue will remain an important challenge to the profession. Similarly, the different but related topic of improved clinical quality is likely to be an issue that new physicians will need to address throughout their careers.

The American Medical Association (AMA) created and sponsors the National Patient Safety Foundation (NPSF), whose website and publications address patient safety concerns. The NPSF also provides research grants for those who may wish to directly expand their knowledge in this area. The Joint Commission for the Accreditation of Healthcare Organizations (JCAHO) has become keenly interested in patient safety as well. A variety of educational materials can be obtained from the JCAHO or from groups that assist in JCAHO accreditation process preparation. A good medically related book on patient safety is Patrice Spath's *Error Reduction in Health Care*.[4] Although not medically related, James Chiles' *Inviting Disaster*[5] is compelling and provides numerous examples of how errors can unexpectedly cascade into disaster. It also examines the various mechanisms of system and human error and how they could have been proactively addressed.

The topic of clinical quality improvement is now commonly encountered in most medical journals. A wonderful overview of the topic can be found in Michael Millenson's *Demanding Medical Excellence*,[6] which provides both a wealth of examples and something of a historical context. The US Department of Health and Human Services' Agency for Healthcare Research and Quality (AHRQ) provides grants for and disseminates findings relating to clinical quality improvement and patient safety. *Research Activities* is published monthly and can either be viewed at their website[7] or may be ordered in hard-copy format free of charge. The provision of brief-synopsis-format reviews of multiple recently published articles and study results makes keeping current in this field far easier.

Important but Neglected

No, this isn't a reference to a preceptor's personal time or spiritual development, but rather to a few items that are often unimportant until the need arises. The first item concerns end-of-life issues. Despite the wish of most individuals to die at home among loved ones, far too many die in institutional settings. This is not only disrespectful of patient wishes but it also imposes an enormous financial burden on a system that is already inefficient. The AMA's Education for Physicians on End-of-life Care (EPEC) project was designed under a grant from the Robert Wood Johnson Foundation. The core curriculum can be ordered from the AMA and includes videotape presentations, or the handbook can be downloaded in PDF format or as PowerPoint slides from the AMA website.[8]

Documentation and coding issues are not commonly emphasized during training. However, given the Office of Inspector General's unwavering interest in fines and costly investigations of a system so complex that even the government's fiscal intermediaries often have different interpretations, it can be a critical skill. Assistance in learning the guidelines can be obtained from various sources, including commercial ones. Local medical societies or State Medical Associations may also have programs or may be able to recommend presenters who have strong track records. The American Health Information Management Association (AHIMA)[9] has produced a wealth of publications and tools relating to coding and related issues.

References

1   www.stfm.org
2   www.nationalahec.org
3   www.aafp.org
4   Spath PL (2000) *Error Reduction in Health Care.* American Hospital Association Press, New York, NY.
5   Chiles JR (2002) *Inviting Disaster.* HarperCollins Publishers, New York, NY.
6   Millenson ML (1999) *Demanding Medical Excellence.* University of Chicago Press, Chicago, IL.
7   www.ahrq.gov
8   www.ama-assn.org
9   www.ahima.org

Chapter 21

Utilizing Electronic Communication and Information Resources

Kate Finkelstein, MLIS

Key Points

- E-mail can be an effective means of communication between residents and preceptors.
- Using electronic information sources can enhance your teaching and patient care.
- The sponsoring institution responsible for the residents may be able to grant you special library privileges, including access to expensive journals and databases.

A recent Harris Poll indicates that 80% of American adults who are online sometimes use the Internet to look for healthcare information.[1] With so many healthcare consumers relying on electronic sources for information, healthcare providers need to be able to access and use the same types of resources. Thanks to the Internet, consumers can search Google and retrieve hundreds of pages of information on any condition. However, most consumers are not equipped with the tools to determine which information is reliable and which is dangerous. In order to better treat and educate their patients, preceptors and residents should become familiar with the resources and services available to them from their university's medical library. In addition, preceptors and residents may learn that e-mail can be a useful tool for sharing information both with each other and with their patients.

E-mail

Because so much medical information is available in the form of electronic journal articles and through online databases, e-mail is a convenient way to share that information among colleagues. Most sponsoring institutions issue a university e-mail account to new residents when they begin their residency. If a preceptor intends to communicate with her residents via e-mail, she should:

1 clarify which e-mail address the resident prefers
2 explicitly inform the resident of her communication expectations.

Although the resident will have an 'official' e-mail address, he may not ever use that account, in which case any mail addressed to that account will go to a 'dead end.' Furthermore, if a resident is not aware that he will receive important information such as scheduling or journal articles via e-mail, he may not check his account as often as the preceptor would like. Therefore the preceptor should clarify these issues early in the preceptor–resident relationship.

Sources of Medical Information

Medical information changes rapidly and so do the avenues of access to that information. In order to stay current with medical science or to locate information related to immediate patient care, the sponsoring institution's library will be the preceptor's best contact. Most sponsoring institutions provide library access to their community preceptors as a benefit of service and as a means of supporting their teaching. These library privileges often include off-campus access to online journals, databases and electronic books. Although a particular preceptor or practice probably cannot afford to subscribe to more than a few of the top medical journals, the sponsoring institution's library can enable the preceptor to use information from many journals. Electronic access means that the preceptor can connect to the library's resources online and can often obtain an article immediately, without having to wait for the article to arrive in the mail and without having to leave the office. The sponsoring institution's library will often also provide links to many useful websites that the library has already evaluated for reliability. The library can be a valuable source of professional information, as well as a place to get helpful information for patients.

Information Management Services

In addition to gaining access to electronic resources, preceptors may enjoy other privileges from the sponsoring institution's library. Many such libraries offer a variety of services to volunteer faculty. These services may include the following.

- Literature Search Service – a librarian will conduct a literature search for the preceptor or resident on a particular topic. The librarian can provide a list of references or can help to answer an immediate question.
- Selective Dissemination of Information (SDI) – a librarian can create an electronic search on a specific topic and run the search monthly. This allows the preceptor to remain up to date with current publications in their field.
- Document Delivery Services – if the library does not hold a particular article that the preceptor needs, the preceptor can usually request the library to obtain that article from another location. Although the preceptor could also request that article directly from a publisher, the library may be able to obtain the article at a lower price and with less time expended on the part of the preceptor.
- Instruction in using library materials – the sponsoring institution's library will often provide classes or consultations for volunteer faculty who want to learn how to search for themselves.

For more information on the information resources available from the sponsoring institution, preceptors should contact the sponsoring institution's library directly.

Electronic communication can be a convenient way for preceptors and residents to share information. As healthcare consumers become more familiar with the use of e-mail and locating health information online, physicians must also learn how to navigate and use electronic medical information. Although a preceptor may recommend that residents rely on the medical literature to provide effective patient care, residents will be more likely to adopt these habits if the preceptor models such behavior himself.

Reference

1   Taylor H (2002) Cyberchondriacs update. In: *The Harris Poll #21, 1 May 2002;* www.harrisinteractive.com/harris_poll/index.asp?PID=299 (accessed 20 June 2003).

Useful Websites

American Academy of Family Physicians; www.aafp.org/
American Academy of Pediatrics: Professional Education; www.aap.org/profed/
American College of Physicians: Products, Programs, and Services to Support and Improve Teaching; www.acponline.org/cme/cbt/faculty.htm
American College of Surgeons: Division of Education; www.facs.org/education/
American Psychiatric Association: Medical Education; www.psych.org/med_ed/
Society of General Internal Medicine: Clinician–Teacher Initiative; www.sgim.org/clinicianteach.cfm
Society of Teachers of Family Medicine; www.stfm.org/

Chapter 22

Costs of Precepting

Brian Finley, MD

> **Key Points**
>
> - The costs of precepting will be most influenced by the experience of the resident and the style of the preceptor.
> - Increasing the frequency and duration of precepting experiences decreases the overall cost.
> - A structured experience will decrease costs.

Precepting residents may have some cost associated with it, but the cost is far outweighed by the benefits for the physician. The main cost is going to be in the extra time (and associated cost of productivity) that it takes to teach and precept. The benefits are enhanced reputation, intellectual stimulation, keeping abreast of new advances in medicine, and the sense of accomplishment that goes with helping to educate the next generation of physicians. When looking for a partner, there is no better way of recruiting than to work with that individual beforehand. There are strategies for addressing cost. Variable factors that influence the cost of precepting include the type of practice, the office where the resident will see the patient, and the resident and the preceptor themselves. The costs of precepting will be most influenced by the experience of the resident and the style of the preceptor.

As with any learning situation, the initial part of a rotation is a time of transition and has a steep learning curve. Once the resident is familiar with your office and patients, you may see the early loss of productivity balanced by later gains. Extending the time of the resident rotation will help to offset the cost to your practice.

The preceptor's style and experience also affect the cost. It has been shown that the more frequently you precept the more efficient you become. Recognition of your own natural style enables you to adjust this style to fit different circumstances and residents. A savvy preceptor can carefully choose how to invest teaching time, electing to closely supervise a resident who is performing a new activity, while allowing more independence when a resident is experienced in performing the procedure.

Time

It will always take time to allow the resident to do something or to teach the resident how to do it. However, keep in mind that in medicine this is the only way to learn, and that someone took the time to teach you. There are various strategies you can use to reduce the cost in terms of time and money.

Strategies for Minimizing Costs

Physicians are experiencing increasing pressure in their clinical practices. With the reduction in reimbursements that we are seeing, it is imperative that we look into and share the ways of balancing the costs of time and money with the benefits of teaching. To keep this cost–benefit ratio favorable, preceptors are encouraged to review the following strategies and explore which ones might be applicable to their clinic, precepting style and residents.

Rewards and Reimbursements

Solicit local hospitals and businesses to support preceptor stipends and residents' room and board. Particularly if you are looking for a new partner, get everyone who will benefit from your new partner to help to defray the cost of having a resident come and work with you. They can be involved with both orientation to medicine in your setting and with the socialization of the resident within the community.

Work with the residents' training program to provide some type of non-monetary rewards. These could include academic appointment, continuing medical educational credit, access to library or Internet resources, training, reduced educational fees for CME, and materials such as medical books or journals.

Resident Orientation and Initial Assessment

- Use clinic staff to help orient and answer residents' questions.
- Orient the resident to the clinic and the staff personnel early and thoroughly.
- Provide your staff and the resident with a written list of expectations and schedules.
- Get to know the resident before you start working with them in clinic. Have them over and get to know their background, experience and skills. Ask them what it is they hope to get out of this experience. Use this information to guide the learning opportunities and adjust the schedule as needed.

Scheduling

- Get schedulers involved early on. Establish beforehand what level of experience the resident has, and then direct those who do your scheduling to create a schedule that will fit the resident's capabilities, skills and preferences.
- Arrive at the office early, and go over the list of patients with the resident to see where any problems might occur and to give the resident insight into any difficult patients.
- Know the rules of what patients you can have the resident see and still be able to see some yourself.

- Experiment and be creative with nontraditional schedule designs (e.g. the wave schedule, alternating with the resident in seeing the patients as they arrive, having the resident see all of the same-day or acute-care visits).
- Build some time into the schedule for catch-up and teaching.
- Increase both the number of residents precepted per year and the length of time that they spend with you. The more you precept the more efficient you will become.
- Schedule residents with other colleagues in the community and have the resident work with each member of your office staff.

Structuring the Patient Encounter

- Have someone screen the resident's patients.
- Depending on the resident's level of experience, directly observe certain patient encounters. Observing how the resident handles particular visits or patients may prevent them from having to present the case, and will give you a better understanding of their capabilities. This technique also provides you with a great source of feedback and teaching points for the resident.
- Maximize teaching in the examining room, educating both resident and patient. This provides residents with role modeling and one-on-one teaching time. It also avoids a lot of repetition due to having to say the same thing to the resident and then to the patient.
- Discuss only issues that are important to the diagnosis and treatment at the time of the visit. Save the more philosophical discussions for after-hours talks and limit the 'war stories' that we all love to tell.

Effective and Efficient Teaching Strategies

- Encourage adult, self-directed learning. Direct the resident to where to look up the information needed for making the diagnosis or deciding on the treatment.
- Have the resident give short updates to your staff (and perhaps you) on new therapies and modalities over the lunch hour.
- Delegate. Assign the resident certain responsibilities. Make them responsible for accomplishing something that you usually have to do. They will learn by having to do it, and you will get back some of the time it takes to teach.
- Allow inexperienced residents to initially observe you performing certain examinations or procedures.
- Maximize opportunities to incorporate teaching tasks into other activities (e.g. driving between clinics or to the hospital, over breakfast or lunch, in meetings).
- Prepare residents to work more efficiently. They must learn how to accommodate their own practice style and incorporate sound time management. Give specific instructions and feedback. Midway through the rotation, ask the resident to evaluate their own progress and develop goals and strategies that they can work on during the last half of the rotation.
- Reframe all daily tasks as potential teaching tools. Modeling how you handle all of the interruptions that occur every day can be educational for the resident.
- Discuss non-medical topics to offer a lesson on how to avoid burnout.

Preceptor Training and Self-Evaluation

- Seek training in teaching and integrating residents into busy practices.
- Learn the skills of time-limited precepting.
- Discuss precepting of residents with your physician and non-physician colleagues. Learn from them how they manage their time and productivity.
- Evaluate your own style and practice flexibility with regard to time management.
- Be aware of your own needs and be sensitive to the resident's needs.

Above everything else, remember that precepting is needed and so are you.

Section III

Teaching at the Next Level

Chapter 23

Getting Formal: Developing a Curriculum for Precepting Medical Residents

Alexander W Chessman, MD

Key Points

- Designing a curriculum involves several key steps, namely needs assessment, objectives, learning activities, and assessment.
- Curriculum design is not linear, but dynamic and interactive.
- Focus your efforts.

There are several reasons for creating a formal curriculum. A well-designed curriculum will help to ensure that residents gain competence in the most important areas. Beyond this outcome, the actual process of creating the curriculum will have positive effects. Clarifying the purpose of your curriculum and its specific learner outcomes often helps you to understand your own values and perfect your own knowledge and skills.

You can build a better relationship with the local residency program by meeting the needs of the program and its residents. Your curriculum may fill an important need for the residency program. For example, the local residency program may have been cited for deficiencies in its geriatrics instruction. In addition, you can develop a better fit between what you and residents expect from the training. Advertising your curriculum accurately will bring you residents whose expectations match the reality of the training that you are interested in providing.

Choose a Focus and Conduct a Needs Assessment

Decide upon a focus for your curriculum. What would you like the curriculum to cover? Let's continue to work through a geriatrics curriculum example. Do not feel that the curriculum must cover everything that you do, even in this area of geriatrics. Choose something specific and small for your first experimentation with curriculum design. For example, suppose that you want to provide excellent training for residents in geriatrics, that you are the medical director of two extended-care facilities, and that you delight in providing family-centered,

93

comprehensive care for your older patients. How do you choose a specific focus within this geriatric care?

Choose something that really interests you, that you do well, and that no one else provides. Conduct a needs assessment, both general and specific. A general needs assessment can use information from the literature. Again, taking the example of geriatrics, cite the statistics about the growing population of Americans who are over 65 or 80 years old. Refer to studies that document residency graduates' poor preparation for caring for this age group. Cite publications that call for improved training in the area as background for your curriculum.

Discuss with the residency director which topics he or she feels are missing or incompletely covered within the residency curriculum. Your passion might match exactly the residency director's programmatic needs. You may have to emphasize a certain aspect of the curriculum so that the residency director will enthusiastically support your offering. For example, the director may have a need for improved practice management, so you build into your curriculum how to bill appropriately for services rendered for older patients who live at home or in an extended-care facility.

The last step in conducting the needs assessment is to discover what the residents actually need. Although the national data and the residency director may emphasize one focus, the residents that you see may already have reasonable competence in that area. There is a natural, recursive process to creating and improving a curriculum. Major adjustments to the objectives often need to be made after the curriculum is in place, and learner outcomes before and after the curriculum have been measured.

Create Goals and Objectives

Once you have conducted the needs assessment and decided upon the focus for your curriculum, you need to decide upon the goals and objectives. To emphasize an earlier point, you don't have to cover everything that the residents will learn. Choose a few key goals and specific learner objectives. Use specific and unambiguous terms. Don't use vague terms such as 'understand', 'appreciate' or 'know.' Use terms like 'define', 'describe' and 'outline' for simpler objectives, and 'demonstrate', 'interpret' and 'justify' for more complex ones.

Some of the objectives can be very specific, giving the context and a measurable outcome for the resident. For example, 'Covering night call for the practice, the resident will accurately determine the best management plan for elders with an acute change in mental status.'

Design Learning Activities

Once you have firmed up your reasons and focus, and created at least a first draft of objectives, you need to design learning activities that will guide the resident through essential experiences. What kinds of activities should be included? This will depend on the learning objectives and on the resources available. It may not be worth having the resident conduct a fully fledged project to improve the system of care by analyzing and changing the admissions process for the nursing home. Instead the learning activities could be as simple as the resident evaluating specific kinds of patients who present to the practice, and conducting certain activities with direct observation and feedback by you. For example, 'The resident will complete one admission history and physical examination per week for the boarding or nursing home.' Maybe you have an objective concerning patient safety and the reduction of error. You might require the resident to interview older patients in different settings (the office, at home, the nursing home) and to discuss with you opportunities for reducing errors and improving patient safety, rather than expecting the resident to change the system, too.

Key features of effective learning activities include clear expectations about the resident's behavior, resources and support to enable the resident to accomplish the tasks well, and opportunities for guided reflection. Make a point of scheduling time to go over the learner's reflections upon the experience. What did they find surprising, difficult and rewarding? How did they feel that they had performed? What did they learn? And how will the resident use the knowledge and skills gained in future care?

Evaluate the Learners and the Program

Your feedback to the resident is critical. There is nothing more powerful than accurate feedback. Presenting feedback so that the learner will accept it is an important skill for any teacher.

Evaluation of the curriculum is helpful. There are different levels of evaluation. The essential question is how well the learner achieved the intended objectives. Feedback from the learner about the program is also helpful.

What did the learner say about the learning activities? Were there some activities that the learners felt were more helpful or enjoyable than others? What else could you change about the curriculum? Did the residents agree with the

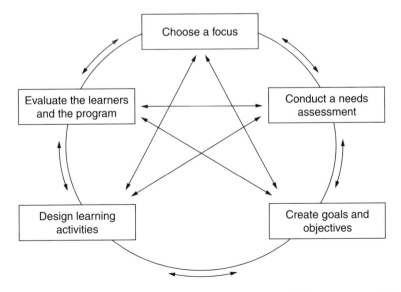

Figure 23.1 Curriculum Development Model. Adapted from Kern *et al.* (1998).[1]

learning objectives? Did the learning activities have some problems with regard to how they were implemented? What would improve the curriculum?

Share the Curriculum with Others

Dissemination of the curriculum is the final step. It can be as simple as sharing the results of learner feedback and accomplishment of learning objectives with the residents who have participated in the program, so that they know and can pass the word on to others that you pay attention to improving their curriculum. Sharing the results with the residency director can help him or her to design a better curriculum that will better prepare the residents to take advantage of your offering.

You may disseminate the results of your work more broadly, at local, regional and national conferences.

The reward of knowing that you are improving the care of hundreds and thousands of patients by helping physicians to gain essential competencies is great. Remember that the needs assessment, objectives, learning activities, and learner and program evaluation do *not* have to be done in any particular order. As you evaluate your curriculum, you will certainly change parts of it, especially the objectives, activities and learner assessment. Pick somewhere to start, and begin there!

Reference

1   Kern DE, Thomas PA, Howard DM and Bass EB (1998) *Curriculum Development for Medical Education. A Six-Step Approach.* Johns Hopkins University Press, Baltimore, MD.

Chapter 24

Getting Trained: Faculty Development

Kent Sheets, PhD

Key Points

- Faculty development can help preceptors to improve their teaching skills.
- Faculty development materials are available in a variety of media.

What Should I Learn?

As a community-based preceptor, you are likely to be interested in the teaching and evaluation skills required to enable you to do an excellent job teaching the residents who are assigned as learners to your practice, or whom you precept in the residents' continuity practice at their residency program site. Other chapters of this book have gone into great detail about the knowledge and skills that will help you to succeed in your role as preceptor concurrently with your successful activities as a physician.

Several sets of preceptor development materials have been used in preceptor workshops throughout the country in recent years, including the Society of Teachers of Family Medicine (STFM) Preceptor Education Project (PEP) materials,[1,2] the Primary Care Futures Project (PCFP) materials[3] and the Teaching in the Ambulatory Setting packaged course.[4] Looking through the table of contents for these materials can give you an idea of what skills you should have as a preceptor.

From the PEP materials, the skills of organization and planning, observation, teaching, feedback, evaluation and handling problems are identified as core precepting skills. A second edition of the PEP materials, PEP2, included the above skills and added the areas of teaching and learning collaboratively and assessment to the PEP2 content.

The PCFP faculty development materials have been used extensively in multi-specialty and multi-disciplinary workshops for faculty in community health centers and other community settings. The PCFP materials emphasize the characteristics of the effective teacher, the components of an educational planning process, different teaching styles and methods, and how to conduct educational evaluation, particularly providing feedback to the learner.

Within the section on the educational planning process, the acronym GNOME is used:

- **G**oals
- **N**eeds of the learner
- **O**bjectives
- **M**ethods of instruction
- **E**valuation.

GNOME reminds the preceptor to consider goals, needs (of the learner), objectives, methods (of instruction) and evaluation during each encounter with the learner. The teaching styles and methods that are proposed are categorized as assertive, suggestive, collaborative and facilitative.

The Teaching in the Ambulatory Setting materials were designed primarily for an internal medicine audience by faculty and staff of the Michigan State University Office of Medical Education Research and Development. The materials cover three major topic areas:

1 planning for the learning encounter
2 teaching in the ambulatory setting
3 evaluating the learning encounter.

David M Irby, PhD has been a pioneer in conducting research on teaching in the ambulatory setting. One of his studies is useful in helping to identify what might be the most critical skills for a community-based teacher.[5] Irby's study was designed to identify the characteristics of clinical teachers in ambulatory care settings that influenced ratings of overall teaching effectiveness. A survey of senior medical students and medicine residents at the University of Washington indicated that the most important characteristics of their ambulatory care teachers were as follows:

1 active involvement of the learners
2 promotion of learner autonomy
3 demonstration of patient care skills.

These results are consistent with those found by other investigators and would suggest that developing and utilizing these teaching behaviors represent the foundation for becoming an outstanding community-based teacher.

Where and How Should I Learn?

There are many sources of preceptor development activities. The secret is to find those that are most accessible to you and compatible with your situation and preferred learning style.

These sources include the following:

1 the residency program or department that sends you residents
2 the residents
3 self-study
4 national and state specialty academy-sponsored activities/materials
5 health system-sponsored activities/materials.

Each of these will be briefly described below.

The Residency Program or Department That Sends You Residents

Your initial source of faculty development in support of your resident teaching should be the residency program or department that assigns residents to work in your practice. Most teaching programs have preceptor manuals or handbooks that outline the basic requirements of you as a preceptor. These manuals often contain faculty development tips or opportunities as well as details of how the resident elective or preceptorship functions.

The residency program or department should also provide regular faculty development via site visits to your practice, workshops on campus or at other locations, and articles or other materials such as the *Family Medicine* column, 'For the Office-Based Teacher of Family Medicine', that many family medicine programs distribute to their preceptors on a regular basis.

States such as North Carolina and Vermont have funded Area Health Education Centers (AHECs), which provide support to community-based preceptors. Examples include the Wake AHEC Office of Regional Primary Care Education (ORPCE) in Raleigh, North Carolina, the Mountain AHEC in Asheville, North Carolina, and the Southern Vermont AHEC in Springfield, Vermont. Preceptors who work in these and other AHEC areas should contact those centers in order to obtain more information on faculty development programs and resources available to them for their teaching activities.

The Residents

The residents assigned to your practice are also a potential source of faculty development. Just as community-based teachers often take advantage of the residents' recent immersion in the academic medical center to learn the latest approach to the treatment of specific diseases, the preceptor can also benefit from the residents' experience with computer and other information technology to improve his or her teaching and self-directed learning skills. Residents can also describe teaching techniques that they have found useful on other rotations, which the preceptor might be encouraged to try as well.

Self-Study

If you get most of your medical CME via self-study methods (audiotapes, journal articles, Internet-based materials, etc.) then you might be likely to use this approach to developing your precepting skills as well. Numerous books, journals and other resources are described in Chapter 20. If you excel at self-directed learning you can develop your skills as a teacher by exploring the various preceptor development materials that are available in print, in various audiovisual media, and in cyberspace.

National and State Academy-Sponsored Activities/Materials

In addition to approaches where physicians learn teaching skills independently or via the residency program or department, there are several avenues for pursuing teaching skill development through national academy-sponsored activities and materials. In addition to specialty-specific organizations such as the American Academy of Family Physicians (AAFP), the American Academy of Pediatrics (AAP) or the American College of Physicians (ACP), there are more broadly based organizations such as the National Health Service Corps (NHSC) and the National Rural Health Association (NRHA) which have incorporated teaching skills sessions into their national meetings or their publications. An example of a publication prepared by a specialty organization is *Community-Based Teaching*, published by the ACP.[6]

The beauty of incorporating teaching skill sessions into these meetings is that it enables physicians to combine their clinical skill development with their teaching skill development in one fell swoop. Within family medicine, each year numbers of your family physician colleagues attend workshops at the AAFP Scientific Assembly in order to develop and enhance their teaching skills. One to two workshops on teaching students and residents in the office are routinely offered as additional workshops at this national meeting.

Several organizations are more geared towards academic physicians, but offer programs or materials for use by the community-based teacher. These include the Society of Teachers of Family Medicine (STFM), the Ambulatory Pediatric Association (APA) and the Society of General Internal Medicine (SGIM). An example of a publication from pediatrics, *Pediatric Education in Community Settings: A Manual*, was published as a joint effort involving the AAP and the APA.[7] Currently the AAP is developing new materials for use by community pediatricians when teaching students and residents. (Check with the AAP for information on how to access the *Starter Kit: A Guide for Pediatricians/ Mentors* and the *Compendium of Resources*, which were made available in 2004 and 2005, respectively.) The STFM provides scholarships for community preceptors to attend some of their national and regional meetings as a means of improving interactions between academic family physicians and their community colleagues.

For some preceptors, there are opportunities at a local and regional level. Some state academies sponsor preceptor development programs as part of state or regional meetings.

In recent years more specialty organizations have made efforts to provide information on faculty development resources on their websites. An Internet search using 'preceptor' as the key word reveals numerous resources that are suitable for self-study. Some resources are developed by the specialty society while others, like the ones mentioned here, are listed on the organization's website.

- The Mountain AHEC in Asheville, North Carolina has online resources at www.mtn.ncahec.org/pdp/preceptors.htm.
- EPIC, the Expert Preceptor Interactive Curriculum from the University of North Carolina, Chapel Hill, is available online at www.med.unc.edu/epic/.
- The University of California-Los Angeles Preceptor Net provides online resources for preceptors at www.medsch.ucla.edu/preceptors/resources.html.

Health System-Sponsored Activities/Materials

In areas of the country where health systems have made a commitment to supporting education, there have been instances where the health system has supported teaching development programs for physicians working at its sites. As more medical schools and residency programs enter into collaborative relationships with health systems, this might become a more frequent source of preceptor development activities.

Summary

There is a wide range of options available to you in your efforts to develop your teaching skills. Your specialty, your geographic location, and the nature of your affiliation with a medical school, residency program and/or health system will dictate some of your options for continued development of your teaching skills. Contact your residency program or department to further explore the options available to you.

References

1 Society of Teachers of Family Medicine (1992) *Preceptor Education Project (PEP) Workshop Materials.* Society of Teachers of Family Medicine, Kansas City, KS.
2 Society of Teachers of Family Medicine (1999) *Preceptor Education Project, Second Edition (PEP2) Workshop Materials.* Society of Teachers of Family Medicine, Kansas City, KS.
3 Massachusetts Statewide AHEC Program (1996) *The Primary Care Futures Project Faculty Development Curriculum. A Multi-Disciplinary Curriculum and Resource Guide for Teaching in Community Health Centers.* Massachusetts Statewide AHEC Program, University of Massachusetts Medical Center, Worcester, MA.
4 Ferenchick G and Langford T (1999) *Teaching in the Ambulatory Setting: a Packaged Course for Physician Teaching Techniques in the Ambulatory Setting.* Michigan State University College of Human Medicine Office of Medical Education Research and Development, East Lansing, MI.
5 Irby DM, Ramsey PG, Gillmore GM and Schaad D (1991) Characteristics of effective clinical teachers of ambulatory care medicine. *Acad Med.* **66:** 54–5.
6 Deutsch SL and Noble J (eds) (1997) *Community-Based Teaching.* American College of Physicians, Philadelphia, PA.
7 DeWitt TG and Roberts KB (eds) (1996) *Pediatric Education in Community Settings: a Manual.* National Center for Education in Maternal and Child Health, Arlington, VA.

Chapter 25

Getting Collegial: Training Across Disciplines

David V O'Dell, MD

Key Points

- Coordinate the resident's schedules to allow the resident to be present during key clinical experiences (i.e. clinics, rounds and conferences).
- Orientation sessions are particularly important for cross-disciplinary rotations.
- Establish a core curriculum and determine the most effective method to cover that curriculum.
- Assess each resident individually and then build knowledge/skills starting at the appropriate level.

Precepting residents from different backgrounds can be a rewarding and enlightening experience and can reinvigorate your own enthusiasm. There are pitfalls, however, although these can be avoided with advance planning and coordination. An essential step is to negotiate with the residency program director the resident's exact schedule during the time when they will be on your rotation. It is particularly frustrating to develop an effective teaching clinic or conference, only to have the resident routinely miss the experience because of their own continuity clinic. Other examples of potential interference include mini-courses (e.g. ACLS, BLS, ATLS, PALS, NALS), obstetrical coverage, moonlighting commitments, licensure exams and vacations. Work to arrange a mutually agreeable schedule and ask the program director to limit outside commitments to agreed exceptions. Once this schedule is in place, as with any clinical experience, flexibility is important, but negotiating a set schedule in advance helps to avoid many problems.

Orientation sessions are essential for all rotations, but are particularly important for cross-disciplinary rotations. These sessions provide an opportunity for introductions and give you the chance to set the tone for the rotation. Take care to avoid overwhelming the resident, and make it clear that they are not expected to be an expert in your area! Reiterate that this is why they are taking the rotation. This approach helps to immediately allay some of the resident's anxiety, and also helps you to build rapport. Provide the resident with written instructions, including call schedules, clinic hours, after-hours coverage, names of key personnel, lists of resources, outlines of how to perform specific tasks (e.g. phone calls/office notes/protocols), and performance expectations.

Keep in mind that residents from different specialties may have time commitments that seem unusual to the preceptor.

Residents from disparate backgrounds will bring with them different skills, knowledge bases and experiences, but all are physicians in training and should be expected to perform as such. Professionalism, work ethic, availability, intellectual curiosity and communication skills should be basic expectations of all residents, regardless of discipline. Residents tend to perform to expectations (a basic human trait), and therefore high expectations should be the rule.

It is critical to assess each resident individually in the context of both the preceptor's and the resident's specialties in order to establish their skills and knowledge. A series of probing questions (i.e. the Socratic method) can be particularly useful for defining the resident's abilities, and this gives you the opportunity to tailor your instruction to the appropriate level. These questions must be asked in a non-threatening manner and the resident must realize that it is OK not to know all the answers. This concept is referred to in the literature as 'psychological safety', and is critical to being an effective cross-disciplinary educator. The task of establishing specific knowledge and ability level is absolutely essential and does require some time and effort, but it helps to avoid many potential problems.

Prioritize the essential concepts in your discipline and then develop a curriculum to cover these topics. This can be as elaborate as time allows, but it may be as simple as a list of the important concepts and a series of articles addressing these topics. A paragon might include a pre-test, a series of lectures, paper/X-ray cases for discussion, clinical conferences discussing actual patient management, structured sessions with support personnel (dietician, physical therapist, nurse educator/coordinator, dialysis technician, etc.), recommended readings, and an appropriate balance between service and education, concluding with a post-test. Determine what is going to work in your situation and then build the necessary infrastructure to support your goals. Some important caveats for residents on rotations outside their area of expertise include the following.

- Focus on common conditions and make it real.
- Stress 'can't-miss diagnoses' (or 'high-impact' conditions) that can result in harm or litigation.
- Keep the curriculum achievable and avoid overwhelming the resident.
- Make the experience as interactive as possible.
- Present a synopsis of the literature and avoid lengthy discussions of all primary studies. Be prepared to discuss the primary literature when specific questions arise.
- Present information in a practical, usable form, including a common work-up and clinical pearls.
- Emphasize where to find timely information (e.g. current guidelines, websites, other resources).
- Remember the role that the resident will be playing in the healthcare system, and put your teaching in that context (e.g. what they can handle and when to refer).

- Stress a screening approach to uncommon conditions, but maintain a focus on common ones.
- Be flexible, and if the clinical workload is excessive, be willing to limit or delay your instruction (remember the 'teachable moment').
- Play 'what if' with the resident's management plan. This allows the resident to think through the plan and possible complications *before* they get the page/call.
- Use residents from different programs to teach each other skills from their areas.

Unusual or rare cases provide an opportunity to assess the resident's judgment and their ability to recognize their own limitations, and reveal their intellectual curiosity. These cases also provide you with the opportunity to model both your own intellectual curiosity and your ability to say 'I don't know.' Use these as teachable moments to emphasize how to deal with uncertainty and the importance of searching the literature. Exposing the resident to 'zebras' is important (you cannot make a diagnosis if you have never heard of it) but should not be unduly emphasized.

Being a good role model is key to being an effective educator. Openly discuss the pros and cons of your discipline and show why you enjoy what you are doing and why it is the 'coolest' job in the world.

Although your basic expectations for all residents should be similar, your final evaluation of the resident should take into account their initial knowledge/skill level, their background, and to some degree the role that they will be playing in the healthcare system. Schedule a face-to-face sit-down evaluation session at the conclusion of the rotation. This allows time to review your written evaluation with the resident, highlighting both their strengths and areas for improvement. Ask them for their thoughts on your rotation. Ask what they thought worked and what didn't, and invite them to make suggestions. Finally, ask them to critique your performance.

No rotation is ever perfect, particularly the first time through, and residents generally sincerely appreciate your time and effort. So don't be intimidated by the thought of allowing residents from other specialties to rotate in your office. Most preceptors find these rotations rewarding on multiple levels. You have much to offer the resident from your personal knowledge to your vast practical experience. In addition to giving back to the profession by helping to train the next generation, residents can be a source of referrals both during residency and once they graduate. This makes the insight they gain from rotating in your practice even more beneficial. Good luck in your efforts!

Acknowledgments

Very little literature has been published on cross-disciplinary precepting of residents, so I chose to elicit additional input from my colleagues at the University of Nebraska, whose teaching is highly regarded by residents from other disciplines. Many of the above suggestions are theirs. I wish to thank Gerald Groggel, MD, Lynell Klassen, MD, Jennifer Larsen, MD, James O'Dell, MD and Joseph Sisson, MD for their willingness to share their time and approaches to training residents from other disciplines.

Further Reading

Alguire AC, DeWitt DE, Pinsky LE and Ferenchick GS (2001) *Teaching in Your Office.* American College of Physicians, Philadelphia, PA.

Edmondson A, Bohmer R and Pisano G (2001) Speeding up team learning. *Harvard Business Rev.* **79:** 125–33.

Irby DM (1995) Teaching and learning in ambulatory care settings: a thematic review of the literature. *Acad Med.* **70:** 898–931.

Sample Resident Affiliation Agreement

THIS AGREEMENT made this _____ day of _____, by and between the Board of Regents of the University governing body for the University Medical Center, hereinafter referred to as 'University' and _____, hereinafter referred to as 'Affiliated Institution.'

Purpose

The common objective of both parties is to provide an educational postgraduate clinical experience for residents in the College of Medicine. The parties agree that the Affiliated Institution will permit a mutually agreed upon number of residents to affiliate with the Affiliated Institution, for a period of time determined by the University, to provide physician services to the Affiliated Institution's patients under the supervision of designated physicians who are members of the active staff of the Affiliated Institution and have been appointed to the teaching faculty of the University.

Term

This agreement is for one year from its effective date.

1 The agreement may be renewed annually by the consent of both parties.
2 Either party may terminate the agreement upon 60 days' prior written notice to the other party provided that no termination shall be effective until completion of the rotation currently in progress at the time the 60 days' notice is given.
3 The parties mutually agree that this written document represents the complete agreement of both parties concerning the terms hereof and that any change in the terms must be contained in writing duly executed by both parties.

Commitments

1 It is mutually agreed by each party that the appropriate 'Institutional' and 'Program' requirements for family practice in Graduate Medical Education as

described in the most current edition of the Essentials of Accredited Residencies in Graduate Medical Education will be met.

2   It is agreed that the University will seek to maintain full accreditation of the residency program by the Accreditation Council for Graduate Medical Education.

Operating Relationships

Program Director

1   Shall be the sole individual selected by the University to be responsible for the residency training program.
2   Will be members in good standing of the medical staff of the Affiliated Institution and will conduct teaching activities within the specific clinical privileges they have granted.
3   Will hold a faculty appointment in the Department.
4   Will be accountable to the program director for the conduct of their teaching assignments.
5   Will conduct their teaching activities within the framework of the Affiliated Institution and medical staff policy.
6   Will evaluate house officer performance in a manner prescribed by the program director and will participate in program evaluation as directed.

House Officers

1   Will be supervised by the teaching staff as designated by the program director.
2   Will be subject to the by-laws, rules and regulations of the Affiliated Institution Medical Staff and to all established policy.
3   Will be assigned in such numbers as agreed upon by the Affiliated Institution and the program director.
4   Will be assigned according to a schedule and for a duration of two months each. The schedule will be developed at least 30 days prior to the beginning of each training year.
5   The assignment of individual house officers may be rejected or terminated by the Affiliated Institution upon notification of the program director by the Affiliated Institution.
6   The appeal of unfavorable evaluation will be in accordance with the procedures outlined in the house officer agreement and the by-laws of the Board of Regents.
7   The Affiliated Institution will provide orientation to the house officer at the beginning of each assignment.

Governance

1   The responsibilities and prerogatives inherent in each of the institutions party to the agreement are recognized.
2   It is understood that the program in Graduate Medical Education will not interfere with the care of the patients at the Affiliated Institution, which

shall remain the primary responsibility of the Affiliated Institution and the medical staff.

3 It is understood that the program in Graduate Medical Education has an obligation to the house officer to provide an educationally rewarding assignment. The determination of such assignments shall be the primary responsibility of the Program Director.

Rights and Responsibilities of the Affiliated Institution

1 Facilities. The Affiliated Institution shall provide reasonable use of such of its facilities as are necessary to provide a high-quality clinical experience.

2 The Affiliated Institution shall retain the right to terminate the use of its facilities, equipment or supplies by any house officer where flagrant or repeated violations of the Affiliated Institution's rules, regulations, and policies or procedures occur. Such action will not normally be taken until the grievance against any house officer has been discussed with the appropriate representative.

3 The Affiliated Institution reserves the right to take immediate action where necessary to maintain operation of its facilities free from interruption.

4 The Affiliated Institution shall furnish lodging for the resident and family for the rotational period. This should be a completely furnished apartment or home.

5 Meals should be supplied for the resident when the practice demands that the resident be at the Affiliated Institution.

6 Each resident will be reimbursed directly for required travel to and from the practice site at a rate of 36.54 cents a mile. This is a one-time reimbursement for each two-month rotation.

7 The administration of the residency training program will be under the direction of the combined family practice residency programs.

8 The Affiliated Institution will be assessed for each two-month residency rotation an amount equivalent to the salary and benefits to that resident for the two months. The total stipend will be paid directly to the Department of Graduate Medical Education, which will distribute these funds to the appropriate residency training program as designated by a related memorandum of understanding.

Rights and Responsibilities of the University

1 The University shall maintain professional liability insurance coverage or self-insurance coverage in the amount of $2,000,000 per occurrence and $600,000 in the annual aggregate and umbrella coverage extending such professional liability coverage to an annual aggregate of not less than $1,250,000 per occurrence and no limit on annual aggregate coverage through a combination of insurance and qualification under and participation in the covering house officers of the University for claims for bodily injury or death on account of alleged malpractice, professional negligence, failure to provide care, breach of contract, or claim based upon failure to obtain informed consent for an operation or treatment. In addition, the University shall maintain professional

liability insurance or self-insurance coverage in the amount of $1,000,000 per occurrence and $3,000,000 in the annual aggregate covering house officers of the University for claims not falling under bodily injury or death on account of alleged malpractice, professional negligence, failure to provide care, breach of contract, or claim based upon failure to obtain informed consent for an operation or treatment.

2   The University is responsible for the academic aspects of the learning experiences of its house officers in all areas of the curriculum.

3   A mutually agreed number of house officers will participate, not exceeding six house officers per year.

4   The University will require its house officers to adhere to the Affiliated Institution's rules, regulations, policies and procedures while on the premises.

5   The house officer is a student/employee of the University and not of the Affiliated Institution. Salaries will be paid to the house officer by the administrative unit of the residency training program.

To the extent permitted by law, both the University and the Affiliated Institution agree to indemnify and hold each other harmless for and against any and all costs, expenses, claims, demands, causes of action, liabilities and responsibilities arising out of or in any way connected with any act or omission of the parties and their respective employees, directors, faculty, house officers, students and/or agents which arises out of the performance of this Agreement.

Equal Opportunity Compliance

Neither the Affiliated Institution nor the University shall discriminate against any employee, applicant or student for employment or registration in its course of study because of race, color, religion, sex, national origin, handicap or Vietnam-era status. Both parties agree to comply with the Educational Rights and Privacy Act of 1974 governing the privacy of house officer records.

in witness whereof the parties hereto have executed this agreement in duplicate upon the first date set forth above:

_____

_____

Chairman, Department of _____

_____ Dean, College of Medicine

_____

_____

Administrator/Physician Affiliated Institution
Vice Chancellor for Finance and
and Business Services

Clinical Teaching Microskills

Get a commitment	'What do you think is going on with this patient?' 'What would you like to do next?' Determine the student's view of the case Don't just ask for more data about the patient Don't immediately provide the answer to the problem
Probe for underlying reasoning	'What led you to that conclusion?' 'What else did you consider and rule out?' Diagnose the learner's understanding of the case gaps in knowledge, poor reasoning or attitudes, and misunderstandings Don't just ask for textbook knowledge
Teach a general rule	'The key features of this illness are ...' The teaching point should help the student to generalize from this case to others Tell the learner what he or she did right. State specifically what was done well and why it is important. This should not be general praise – be specific
Correct errors	'Next time this happens, try this ...' Make recommendations for improvement; be future oriented. Uncorrected errors may be repeated

Reprinted with permission from Neher JO, Gordon KC, Meyer B and Stevens N (1992) A five-step 'microskills' model of clinical teaching. *J Am Board Fam Pract.* **5**: 419–24.

Index

Page numbers in *italic* refer to tables and figures.